G000126182

BACTERIOLOGY RESEARCH DEVELOPMENTS

BACTEREMIA

RISK FACTORS, TREATMENT AND POTENTIAL COMPLICATIONS

BACTERIOLOGY RESEARCH DEVELOPMENTS

Additional books in this series can be found on Nova's website under the Series tab.

Additional e-books in this series can be found on Nova's website under the e-book tab.

BACTERIOLOGY RESEARCH DEVELOPMENTS

BACTEREMIA

RISK FACTORS, TREATMENT AND POTENTIAL COMPLICATIONS

JODIE P. WILLIAMS
EDITOR

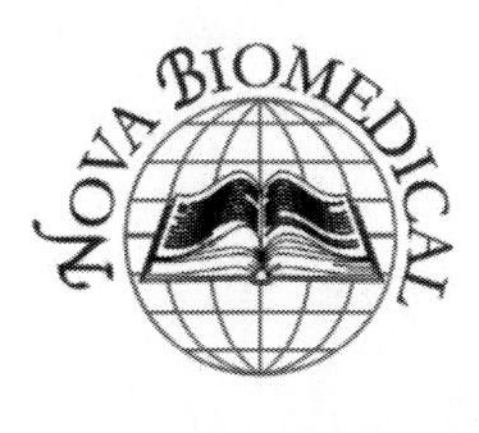

New York

For permission to use material from this book please contact us:
Telephone 631-231-7269; Fax 631-231-8175
Web Site: http://www.novapublishers.com

Library of Congress Cataloging-in-Publication Data

ISBN: 978-1-63117-290-8

Library of Congress Control Number: 2014931437

Published by Nova Science Publishers, Inc. † New York

Contents

Preface

Expert Committees have developed antimicrobial protocols for the prevention of potential complications derived from bacteremia of oral origin, such as infective endocarditis. These preventive protocols have subsequently been revised and modified based on the extensive research that has been performed in this field, including studies on the efficacy of antimicrobial prophylaxis in the prevention of bacteremia of oral origin. This book provides insight on the potential implications of bacteremia of oral origin, and prevention of these potential implications with antibiotics and antiseptics. The book also discusses a rare cause of bateremia known as Lactobacillemia.

Chapter I - The human oral cavity harbors a wide array of different bacterial species (>100 bacterial genera and >700 species). Most of these bacterial species are thought to be of a commensal nature, engaging in complex biofilm formation and facilitating the colonization of more noxious and pathogenic bacteria. Oral bacteria are the main infectious cause of two of the most endemic and historic diseases known to man: dental caries and periodontal disease. A number of unique characteristics of the mouth such as higher temperature, permanent humidity, a variety of substrate surfaces for attachment (teeth, tongue, cheeks and other oral soft-tissue surfaces) and decreased oxygen tension facilitate the formation of a biofilm that continuously challenges the host mucosal immune system. When undisturbed, mature oral microbial communities are formed. These are largely anaerobic Gram-negative bacteria under the gum-line and facultative gram-positive bacteria above the gum-line. Oral microbial communities ultimately overwhelm the local immune response and facilitate local infection. Epithelial cells, endothelial cells, take up the microorganisms and their antigens and innate immune cells, leading to immune dysregulation. With no obvious clinical signs or symptoms experienced by the infected individual, a long-standing chronic oral inflammatory response develops and ultimately progresses to a systemic inflammation stage. During disease development, translocation of oral bacteria to the bloodstream, i.e., bacteremia, ensues, modifying immune homeostasis in the process. This results in continued systemic infection and inflammation with potential systemic consequences. This chapter will focus on reviewing the current evidence of bacteremias of oral origin and how they affect different systems. Human evidence as well as experimental evidence obtained from *in vitro* and *in vivo* studies will be discussed to explain the potential implications to other systemic diseases.

Chapter II - Lactobacillemia is a rare cause of bacteremia and the true clinical significance of this entity is just being delineated. *Lactobacillus* is a gram-positive bacillus that is for the most part intrinsically resistant to vancomycin but appears to be susceptible to most beta-lactams, erythromycin and clindamycin. *Lactobacilli* are a part of the normal gastrointestinal and genitourinary flora and for many years was regarded as non-pathogenic. There have been several case reports of *Lactobacillus* causing infections such as bacteremia, abscesses, peritonitis, meningitis and endocarditis.

L. rhamonosus, L. acidophilus and *L. casei* seem to have been implicated in a variety of infections. Interestingly, pre-administration of commercially available probiotics seem to have been implicated in sepsis in some of these cases. Lactobacillemia may be seen as an isolated infection or more often, as a poly-microbial infection. It tends to occur in patients who have been treated with antibiotics that have no activity on *Lactobacillus.* Many of the patients described in the literature are immuno-compromised with underling disease processes such as cancer, recent surgery, diabetes, and immunosuppressive therapy. However, patients with normal immune systems and *Lactobacillus* infection have also been described in the literature. Diagnosis is usually made on the isolation of the pathogens on blood cultures but more recently can be made using a rapid molecular method using terminal restriction fragment polymorphism analysis of the 16S rRNA gene. Some interesting questions still remain to be addressed such as recommendations in the use of prophylactic *Lactobacillus* on diseases such as irritable bowel syndrome, *Clostridium difficile* colitis and even routine use of this supplement and the risk of bacteremia.

Chapter III - Expert Committees have developed antimicrobial protocols for the prevention of potential complications derived from bacteremia of oral origin, such as infective endocarditis. These preventive protocols have subsequently been revised and modified based on the extensive research that has been performed in this field, including studies on the efficacy of antimicrobial prophylaxis in the prevention of bacteremia of oral origin. The aim of this chapter is to provide an overview of existing studies about bacteremia secondary to dental procedures in humans, showing results concerning the efficacy of both antibiotic and antiseptic prophylaxis, as well as presenting which are the most studied active principles, their doses or concentrations, time and route of administration or the application technique.

The prevention of bacteremia of oral origin has mostly focused on the use of antibiotic prophylaxis prior to dental extractions. However, there are important differences with respect to the type and dose of antibiotic used and time of administration. Penicillins have been the most-studied antibiotics for bacteremia prophylaxis both by oral and parenteral routes. The doses and time of administration varied from 1–3 g and 1–2 hours, respectively, for the oral route which has been the most-studied route of administration. Clindamycin, azithromycin and cephalosporin have been posed as alternatives in allergic patients, although fewer studies exist concerning their prophylactic efficacy.

Some Expert Committees have recommended another complementary method for the prevention of bacteremia of oral origin, which is antiseptic prophylaxis. Numerous reports exist concerning the efficacy of antiseptics at preventing bacteremia secondary to dental procedures. However, there are significant methodological differences related to the dental treatment, the type of antiseptic used and its concentration, as well as the application technique of the antiseptic solution (mouthwash, toothbrush and/or irrigation). The mouthwashes, performed individually or in combination with irrigation, have been the most-studied application technique. Regarding the antiseptic protocol, chlorhexidine has been the most-tested antimicrobial agent, although povidone iodine and essential oils appear to be possible options. However, none of them has been demonstrated to be clearly effective at reducing bacteremia secondary to dental procedures.

Nowadays, the controversies concerning the efficacy of antibiotic prophylaxis and the risk/cost-benefit relationships of antibiotic prophylaxis might justify the convenience of more extensive research on the recommended chlorhexidine regimens and new antiseptic protocols, specifically analysing their effect on the magnitude and duration of bacteremia of oral origin.

In general terms, further evidence-based well-designed research on the efficacy of antimicrobials in the prevention of oral bacteraemic episodes is needed. This is in order to reach a major consensus in the scientific community on the antimicrobial prophylaxis of potential complications, derived from a bacteremia of oral origin.

Chapter IV - Bacterial sepsis is a frequent occurrence during the first 1–2 months after liver transplantation under immunosuppressive therapy. Despite recent advances in perioperative management and surgical techniques, postoperative mortality and morbidity rates are still associated with infectious complications, such as bacterial sepsis, after liver transplantation. Furthermore, bacterial sepsis is the most frequent cause of in-hospital death after living donor liver transplantation (LDLT).

In this chapter, the etiology, outcomes, and risk factors of bacterial sepsis after LDLT are discussed. In addition, we focus on the effect of perioperative nutritional support in LDLT for preventing bacterial sepsis after LDLT. LDLT involves a smaller graft size and scheduled non-emergent surgery compared with deceased donor liver transplantation. A smaller graft size is the main disadvantage of adult-to-adult LDLT because it results in increased portal venous pressure, impaired bowel motility, bacterial translocation, ascites production, and hyperbilirubinemia.

In the last 2 decades, nutritional support has been recognized as a vital component for the management of critically ill patients, by delivering preoperative essential substrates and nutrition using enteral feeding, to aid patient recovery. In particular, preoperative branched-chain amino acid supplementation might reduce the incidence of postoperative bacterial sepsis after LDLT. Additionally, early enteral nutrition is associated with a significantly reduced risk of developing bacterial sepsis after LDLT.

Therefore, poor nutritional status of pre-transplants can be improved by using nutritional support, and the high infectious status of post-transplants under immunosuppressive therapy can be improved with initiation of early postoperative enteral nutrition. Improved nutrition supports a functional immune system, and reduces septic morbidity and mortality in patients with liver transplantation.

In: Bacteremia
Editor: Jodie P. Williams

ISBN: 978-1-63117-290-8

Chapter I

Bacteremias of Oral Origin and Potential Implications for Systemic Diseases

R. M. Arce and C. W. Cutler
Department of Periodontics, Georgia Regents University – College of Dental Medicine, Augusta, GA, US

Abstract

The human oral cavity harbors a wide array of different bacterial species (>100 bacterial genera and >700 species). Most of these bacterial species are thought to be of a commensal nature, engaging in complex biofilm formation and facilitating the colonization of more noxious and pathogenic bacteria. Oral bacteria are the main infectious cause of two of the most endemic and historic diseases known to man: dental caries and periodontal disease. A number of unique characteristics of the mouth such as higher temperature, permanent humidity, a variety of substrate surfaces for attachment (teeth, tongue, cheeks and other oral soft-tissue surfaces) and decreased oxygen tension facilitate the formation of a biofilm that continuously challenges the host mucosal immune system. When undisturbed, mature oral microbial communities are formed. These are largely anaerobic Gram-negative bacteria under the gum-line and facultative gram-positive bacteria above the gum-line. Oral microbial communities ultimately overwhelm the local immune response and facilitate local infection. Epithelial cells, endothelial cells, take up the microorganisms and their antigens and innate immune cells, leading to immune dysregulation. With no obvious clinical signs or symptoms experienced by the infected individual, a long-standing chronic oral inflammatory response develops and ultimately progresses to a systemic inflammation stage. During disease development, translocation of oral bacteria to the bloodstream, i.e., bacteremia, ensues, modifying immune homeostasis in the process. This results in continued systemic infection and inflammation with potential systemic consequences. This chapter will focus on reviewing the current evidence of bacteremias of oral origin and how they affect different systems. Human evidence as well as experimental evidence obtained from *in vitro* and *in vivo* studies will be discussed to explain the potential implications to other systemic diseases.

Background

Human teeth have been linked to infection and pain for ages. Archaeological findings from the bone and teeth of long-dead humans have identified evidence of dental problems going back thousands of years. Even Hippocrates, who is considered the 'father of medicine', reported a case of an arthritis patient that was cured by means of a tooth extraction in ancient Greece. Nonetheless, the specific role of infection in tooth pain was not identified until modern medicine arrived. The landmark establishment of Koch's postulates defined the causal relation between microbes and diseases in the late 19th century.

Circa this period, the German physician Willoughby Miller specifically linked oral diseases to medical infections, giving birth to the theory of focal infection. The theory of focal infection hypothesized that a local infection confined to a small area of the body can ultimately lead to other infection(s) in different parts of the body because of infective agent and/or toxin spreading. Consequently, the mouth was proposed as a classical localized infection site exemplifying the concept of focal infection. Physicians in the early 20th century strongly believed that oral sepsis was the cause of gastritis, neural disorders, meningitis, endocarditis, osteomyelitis and other septic conditions [1, 2]. In fact, during the 1920-30's the theory of focal infection gained so much popularity that dentists pulled many teeth unnecessarily, mostly because dentists were following physicians' instructions. This approach ultimately was recognized to be flawed by both medical and dental communities; moreover, with the development of dental x-ray technology, dentists promoted oral disinfection, conservative restorative dentistry, endodontic (root canal) therapy and preservation of oral health. Overall these developments hastened the disregard of focal infection theory by the 1950's [3].

Regardless of this development, the focal infection theory persists with more recent evidence supporting the oral cavity as a unique site of infection with systemic disease implications that are plausible; moreover, it helped to unify the concept of oral health and primary care integration [4]. To date, a considerable amount of scientific literature has addressed the role of oral infections (such as periodontal disease) in the pathogenesis of medical problems such as atherosclerotic cardiovascular disease, diabetes, obesity, respiratory infections and adverse pregnancy outcomes.

Though still controversial in many aspects, a number of plausible biological mechanisms have been proposed that could explain the link between periodontal infection and systemic diseases. One common biological mechanism relates to the ability of oral bacteria to evade the innate and adaptive immune responses and translocate to other body compartments by means of transient and periodic episodes of asymptomatic bacteremia.

In this chapter we will begin with a discussion of the current general concepts of oral microbiology, define the role of mucosal immunity in the interaction with key oral pathogens, and present the scientific evidence supporting bacteremias of oral origin. This will be followed by review of the interactions of oral pathogens with organ systems and the potential implications for systemic diseases.

Oral Microbiology: From Colonization and Microbial Biofilm Complexes to "Keystone" Pathogens

The oral cavity harbors more than 700 bacterial species or phylotypes, and over 50% of these bacteria have not yet been cultivated [5]. As most of the microbial biomass on earth grows attached to surfaces, oral planktonic bacteria find oral surfaces (namely mucosal tissues and teeth) as ideal surfaces for attachment, growth and survival. A wide variety of different surfaces (keratinized/non-keratinized epithelium, dental enamel, cementum, calculus) and topographies (cratered tongue/tonsils, smooth mucosal linings) facilitate bacterial colonization and spreading [6].

Most oral bacteria are considered "normal" flora of a relatively benign nature. However, there are significant microbial profile changes when the ecological balance between the host and the microbe is disrupted, favoring the recruitment of more 'toxic' species. For example, >140 different bacterial taxa including Firmicutes (*Streptococcus*, *Gemella*, *Eubacterium*, *Selenomonas*, *Veillonella*), Actinobacteria (*Actinomyces*, *Atopobium*, *Rothia*), Proteobacteria (*Neisseria*, *Eikenella*, *Campylobacter*), Bacteroidetes (*Porphyromonas*, *Prevotella*, *Capnocytophaga*), Fusobacteria (*Fusobacterium* and *Leptotrichia*), and the TM7 phylum (no cultivable representatives) have been identified in apparently healthy oral conditions [5]. In dental caries, the number of bacterial species increases to up to 224 species with about 60% being not-yet-cultivable phylotypes [7]. In periodontal disease, the number rises to 200-400 microorganisms in the subgingival environment [8, 9].

Specific oral bacteria preferentially colonize different oral cavity surfaces as a result of specific virulence factors (e.g. adhesins) that bind to complementary substrate-specific receptors on any given oral surface like mucosa or teeth. However, bacterial attachment is not sufficient for growth and survival, so oral bacteria 'engineer' the development of complex microbial communities seeking for mutualism and synergy with other more pathogenic oral bacteria. This phenomenon is known as biofilm formation. The term biofilm was coined in the 70's to describe relatively indefinable microbial communities associated with a tooth surface or any other hard non-shedding material, randomly distributed in a shaped matrix or glycocalyx [10]. For example, microorganisms contained in a mature dental plaque biofilm over teeth surfaces are estimated to be close to 10^9 bacteria per gram with up to 200 different microbial phylotypes [11].

The establishment of a sequential biofilm formation is essential for microbial growth and survival in the human oral cavity [12]. Initially, select *Streptococcus* species adhere to oral epithelial surfaces or teeth, often aided by saliva or sucrose-rich substrates [13]. An example of one of these "pioneer" species is S. *gordonii,* which attach to the salivary pellicle that coats exposed teeth surfaces, along with other *Actinomyces* spp. These are generally also known as early colonizers, and are considered of commensal nature at least in their preferred niche. Later, as the biofilm matures, more microbial interactions between early and intermediate/late colonizers occurs. Late colonizers such as *Fusobacterium nucleatum*, *Tannerella forsythia*, *Treponema denticola* and *Porphyromonas gingivalis* are incorporated into a more mature form of a dental biofilm, rich in exopolysaccharides (sugar-rich residues), fluid channels and quorum-sensing molecules [10]. The maturation process of the dental biofilm is believed to be closely associated with a more pathogenic role in caries and periodontal disease. For example, the early colonizer *Streptococcus mutans* can ferment carbohydrates to produce lactic acid, lowering the oral pH to acidic levels that lead to tooth enamel demineralization and dental caries [14]. In the case of periodontal pathogens, most of which are obligate anaerobes, biofilm maturation confers ideal conditions for them to thrive; facilitated by periodontal disease progression, the subgingival environment becomes colonized with these anaerobes facilitating biofilm progression, bacterial growth and host invasion. This process is aided local inflammation culminating in alveolar bone loss [15].

To recap, dental plaque is a complex and dynamic biofilm that develops mostly on non-shedding tooth surfaces by means of sequential and ordered accumulation of several hundred species of cultivable and non-cultivable oral bacteria [16]. The concept of ordered colonization by early, intermediate and late colonizers consisting of different groups of bacteria gained momentum in the last twenty years due to advances in molecular DNA hybridization and sequencing. Specific bacterial associations have been found to 'cluster' during biofilm formation and maturation. These clusters were denoted as 'bacterial complexes' [17]. For didactic purposes, these bacterial complexes were given color designations (i.e., green, yellow, blue, purple, orange and red) to illustrate a sequential order of colonization leading to periodontal disease [18]. Most complexes included commensal and pathogenic bacteria, but the 'red' complex consists of three late-colonizers, *Porphyromonas gingivalis* (Pg), *Tannerella forsythia* (Tf) and *Treponema denticola* (Td). *These* were proposed as the most pathogenic species in the development of periodontal disease as a result of microbiological and clinical results from periodontitis patients and healthy controls around the globe [19].

More recent thinking has proposed the theory that infectious oral diseases are the result of a 'dysbiotic' biofilm rather than the direct effect of red complex bacteria on the host [20]. This new concept proposes that microbial synergy among biofilm colonizers shape and stabilize a disease-provoking microbial profile that disrupts equilibrium with the host, leading to a diseased state. Several lines of evidence, mostly centered on the known periodontopathogen *P. gingivalis*, support this theory. *P. gingivalis* is not a potent standalone inducer of inflammation and often-contradictory responses to Pg are observed in *in vitro* and *in vivo* animal studies. For example, *P. gingivalis* LPS can antagonize toll-like receptor 4 unlike other highly pro-inflammatory LPS from most Gram negative bacteria [21]. In the absence of commensal bacteria *P. gingivalis* fails to induce periodontitis when used as a mono-infection in germ-free mice [22]. The theory is that *P. gingivalis* is a keystone pathogen that can elevate the pathogenicity of commensal bacteria within the biofilm by disrupting host-bacterial homeostasis [20].

Oral Mucosal Immunity: When Too Much Becomes Detrimental

The human mouth is considered an immuno-privileged body compartment, mainly based on a complex mucosal (and secretory) immune system. The mouth is rich in mucosa-associated lymphoid tissue (MALT) that covers the complete digestive tract, with the mouth being the portal of entry. The gingiva around teeth, the tonsils and adenoids in the nasal cavity or Peyer's patches in the small intestine are examples of MALT associated structures. Also, mucosal secretions and salivary gland products form the saliva, flushing away bacteria from surfaces as well as carrying secretory immunoglobulin A that acts as a potent antimicrobial that can survive harsh environments (such as digestive and respiratory tracts). Also, gingival crevicular fluid (GCF) is a tissue transudate that flows from the gingiva through the epithelial seal to wash out bacterial accumulation in the subgingival environment. Despite this, bacteria largely attach to oral surfaces, with the number of bacteria colonizing mucosal and skin surfaces exceeding the number of host cells that form the human body. Outnumbered, the host has evolved a number of protective mechanisms to tolerate commensal bacteria but resist the invasion of pathogens. However, under specific conditions the host is unable to maintain protective host responses and ultimately suffers from pathologic effects [23].

The first line of host immune response in the mouth is the innate defense system. Epithelial cells represent the 'soldiers on the front line' of this interface. Accordingly, epithelial cells have evolved the ability to recognize pathogenic from harmless bacteria (microbial components or antigens) by expression of pattern recognition receptors (PRRs) that mediate the recognition of structures and process this information by activating intracellular signaling pathways. An example is the Toll-like receptors (TLRs), which enable most mammalian cells to recognize conserved characteristic molecules on microorganisms. These molecules are generally termed as pathogen-associated molecular patterns (PAMPs). Different TLRs bind to different PAMPs, which include lipopolysaccharide (LPS), peptidoglycans, lipoteichoic acid, flagellin, double-stranded viral RNA and unmethylated bacterial DNA and among others [24]. This confers some specificity to the innate immune response, heretofore through to be non-specific. Thus epithelial cells are not passive bystanders rather are metabolically active and capable of reacting to different external stimuli by synthesizing a number of antimicrobial peptides (defensins), cytokines (IL-8), adhesion molecules (epCAM), growth factors (EGF) and enzymes (pepsin) [25].

Despite the key role of epithelial cells in innate immunity, microorganisms can overcome the epithelial defense by means of cell invasion and immune evasion. For example, there is good evidence to support invasion of epithelial cells and fibroblasts by a number of subgingival bacteria [26]. This mechanism provides a shelter effect from the host defenses, and it is also believed to drive the release of other pro-inflammatory cytokines, which turn on a vascular response and lead to inflammatory events [25].

In the case of periodontal disease pathogenesis, invading microbial agents and their virulence factors trigger the disease process. As the host responds to these ‘danger signals’ by activating a cascade of molecular signals that disrupt local immune homeostasis, the net result is local inflammation and ultimately ‘collateral tissue damage’ (i.e., alveolar bone loss) [27]. A wide array of cytokines, chemokines, arachidonic acid metabolites and proteolytic enzymes play crucial roles in initiating the complex disease process. Briefly, interleukin 8 (IL-8) produced by the epithelial cells increases polymorphonuclear leukocytes (PMNs) recruitment and migration to the infected periodontal tissue in response to bacterial infection (acting as a chemokine). Virulence factors such as LPS stimulate neutrophils and mast cells to release vasoactive peptides (via tumor necrosis factor - TNFα) and cause a release of inflammatory mediators in resident cells of the gingival tissue (fibroblasts) and invading immune cells. This ‘amplifies’ the local immune response, as PMNs and myeloid inflammatory cells are increasingly recruited via diapedesis and facilitated by vasodilation. PMNs continue to release lysosomal enzymes in an effort to control the local challenge, but also lead to collagen degradation of the gingival tissue by activating matrix metalloproteinases (MMPs) and altering connective tissue homeostasis [25]. The uncontrolled process leads to the recruitment of lymphocytes and macrophages. As innate immunity links to acquired immunity, antigen-presenting cells (such as dendritic cells – DCs) activate Th0 cell and lead to Th1, Th2 or Th17 T cell effector responses. These in turn can increase or decrease the production of inflammatory mediators as the disease becomes chronic and undergoes periods of activation and remission [28].

Table 1. Sites of oral bacteria translocation and potential pathogenesis implications in humans*

Oral genus (*spp*)	Blood (bacteremia)	Cardiovascular	Fetoplacental unit	GI tract	Rheumatoid arthritis/Autoimmune conditions	Non-Oral Abscesses in the body
Porphyromonas (*gingivalis*)	Chronic PD patients [DNA: [50, 56, 173, 174], culture: [51]] RA patients [DNA: [143, 175]	Atheromatous plaque [DNA: [28, 29, 176], histology: [71]]; Thrombus aspirates [DNA: [177]]	Placenta [histology: [98], DNA: [178, 179]]; Amniotic Fluid [DNA: [100, 180]]	Gastric pre-cancerous lesions [DNA: [130]]; Colorectal cancer biopsies [RNA: [127]]	Synovial fluid [DNA: [139, 143], IgG antibodies§: [140]]	Pyogenic liver abscess [histology: [156]]; Perirectal abscesses [culture: [167]]
Aggregatibacter (*actinomycetem comitans*)	Chronic PD patients [DNA: [50]	Atheromatous plaque [DNA: [29, 176], histology: [71]]; Infective endocarditis [DNA: [181]]; Thrombus aspirates [DNA: [177]]; Valves (aortic, mitral) [DNA: [182]]	Placenta [DNA: [179]]; Preeclampsia [culture and DNA: [99]]	Gastric pre-cancerous lesions [DNA: [130]]	Serum (IgG) antibodies§: [183]	Brain abscesses [DNA:[157], culture: [184]]
Tannerella (*forsythia*)	Chronic PD patients [culture: [51]]; RA patients [DNA: [139, 143]]	Atheromatous plaque [DNA: [28, 29], histology: [71]]	Amniotic fluid [DNA: [180]]; Preeclampsia [culture and DNA: [99]]	IBD [DNA: [128]]	Synovial fluid [DNA: [139]]	Brain abscesses [RNA: [185]]
Treponema (*denticola*)	RA patients [DNA: [143]]	Thrombus aspirates [DNA: [177]]; Valves (aortic, mitral) [DNA:[182]]; Atheromatous plaque [DNA:[186];	Placenta [DNA: [178, 179]]; Preeclampsia [culture and DNA: [99]]	Gastric pre-cancerous lesions [DNA: [130]]	NR	Pyogenic liver abscess [histology: [156]]
Eikenella (*corrodens*)	Chronic PD patients [culture: [51]]	Atheromatous plaque [DNA: [20]]	Placenta [culture:[105]	Appendicitis [culture: [169]] Bowel carcinoid tumor [culture: [187]]	NR	Intraperitoneal abscess [culture: [168]]; Appendicitis [culture: [169]]
Fusobacterium (*nucleatum*)	Chronic PD patients [culture: [51]]	Atheromatous plaque [DNA: [28, 29], Histology:[71]]	Amniotic fluid [culture: [103], DNA: [188, 189]]; Placenta [DNA: [179], culture: [104]]; Stillbirth [culture: [190]]	Colorectal carcinoma biopsies [RNA: [133], DNA: [134]]; IBD patients (culture: [191]]	Failed prosthetic joints [DNA: [192]]	Brain abscess [DNA: [103, 194]]; Appendicitis [RNA: [171]]

Oral genus (*spp*)	**Blood (bacteremia)**	**Cardiovascular**	**Fetoplacental unit**	**GI tract**	**Rheumatoid arthritis/Autoimmune conditions**	**Non-Oral Abscesses in the body**
Campylobacter (*rectus*)	Chronic PD patients [culture: [51]]	Atheromatous plaque [DNA: [29]]	Amniotic fluid [DNA: [180]]; Fetal cord blood§ [fetal IgM antibodies: [107]]	IBD patients [culture and DNA:[195]];	Synovial fluid [RNA: [141]]	Brain abscess [DNA: [193]]
Prevotella (*intermedia*)	Chronic PD [culture:[196]]; RA patients [DNA: [143]]	Atheromatous plaque [DNA: [176. 197], histology:[71]]; Valves (aortic, mitral) [DNA:[182]	Placenta [DNA: [179]]; Preeclampsia [culture and DNA:[99]]	Crohn's disease biopsies [DNA: [198]]	Synovial fluid [DNA: [139, 143]]	Pyogenic liver abscess [histology:[156]]
Streptococci (*mitis, mutants, sanguinis, viridans, parasanguis*)	Chronic PD patients [DNA and culture: [196, 199]; After dental extractions [culture: [199-201]];	Valves (aortic, mitral) [DNA:[182]	Amniotic fluid [culture: [202]]	Ileostomies [RNA: [203]]	Synovial fluid [RNA:[142]], neutropenic patients [RNA:[204]]	Congenital coronary arteriovenous fistula [culture:[205]]; Brain abscess [RNA:[206]]

*Relevant literature examples have been included for illustration purposes, however several references were unintentionally excluded due to space limitations.

§Indirect evidence via specific immunoglobulin G or M (IgG or IgM).

PD= Periodontal disease; IBD=inflammatory bowel disease; NR=Not reported/not found.

When exacerbated, pro-inflammatory cytokines such as IL-1 β, IL-6 and prostaglandins E2 (PGE2) affect bone metabolism by activating anabolic pathways; in particular, receptor activator of nuclear factor-κB ligand (RANKL) leads to the formation and activation of osteoclasts capable of alveolar bone degradation around teeth. When untreated, the disease drives alveolar bone loss leading to tooth loss, but also sustains the host into a pro-inflammatory state for decades [29].

Oral Bacteremias: Casual Dissemination or Targeted Effects?

Because of the nature of oral biofilm infections, the interaction between host and pathogens in the mouth and the subsequent chronic nature of oral infections, it is not surprising to find that oral bacteria are capable of entering the bloodstream of humans. Several publications validate bacteremias originated from the mouth, as oral bacteria are frequently found in blood as well as in distant remote sites associated with different body tissues (Table 1). However, one of the biggest conundrums in dental research is the actual clinical and pathophysiological significance of dissemination of oral bacteria into the bloodstream.

In fact, random transient bacteremias of oral origin do occur after physiological processes like mastication, or after oral hygiene practices like tooth brushing, flossing/wooden cleansing devices [30]. Bacteremias also occur during and/or after conventional dental treatments like dental prophylaxis (conventional cleaning), scaling and root planning (biofilm removal in periodontitis patients), tooth extractions (exodontia) and periodontal surgery (open flap debridement). The frequency of oral bacteremia episodes has been reported with an ample variation of 3-100% [31-34].

The majority of dental/medical community members recognize a severe potential outcome of oral bacteremia: infective endocarditis (IE). IE is an infection of the endocardial surface of the heart, which may include one (or more) heart valves, the mural endocardium, or a congenital septal defect. The detrimental consequences of IE include several intracardiac effects like severe valvular insufficiency, congestive heart failure and myocardial abscesses. Although IE incidence is rare (2-6 cases/100.000 people/years) [35], IE is generally fatal if left untreated. Streptococci from the oral cavity have been implicated in between 35-45% and even up to 65% of IE cases, and it is generally believed that dental procedures significantly increase the risk of bacteremia potentially leading to IE [36].

To address IE risk, guidelines from the American Heart Association and the American Dental Association have been developed for medical and dental practitioners to use antibiotic prophylaxis for the prevention of IE since 1955 [37]. To date, 9 guidelines have been generated, varying greatly based on patient selection, antibiotic selection and dosing schemes [38]. The issue of antibiotic prophylaxis in dental procedures to reduce IE risk has become increasingly controversial mostly due to the lack of high-evidence data coming from randomized clinical trials, the biological complexity of the disease and the relatively low frequency of IE in different populations [39. 40]. In fact, countries like the UK have abolished the use of antibiotic prophylaxis in their guidelines for dental procedures, and have recently reported no effects in the prevalence of IE cases after 2 years of implementation [41, 46]. Although invasive dental procedures may facilitate the entrance of oral bacteria into circulation, there is also evidence that transient bacteremia with oral organisms occurs during conventional daily activities as discussed above. Nonetheless, it is believed that the bacterial load and frequency of the oral bacteremia is significantly greater in patients with abundant biofilm plaque and poor oral hygiene [34], so optimal hygiene and oral health maintenance maybe more important than antibiotic prophylaxis for the majority of patients. There are however some patients with cardiac conditions (such as patients with prosthetic valve replacements or congenital heart disease defects) in whom antibiotic prophylaxis maybe reasonably beneficial [39].

Despite the controversy, the reality is that whether these bacteremias cause significant enough bacterial load to initiate a focal infection in other body compartments is currently unknown. Evidence from animal models suggests that high-level bacteremias are not required to induce experimental endocarditis and rather supports the hypothesis that cumulative exposure to low-grade bacteremia represents a genuine risk for IE [42]. Furthermore, patients' susceptibility to oral bacteremias may also vary significantly. Oral bacteremia episodes occurs on multiple occasions; moreover, over 1 year the cumulative everyday-risk of bacteremia is nearly 6 million times higher than a bacteremia experienced from a dental extraction [43]. In some cases, some patients may "tolerate" these bacteremias while others might be more susceptible and prone to develop other systemic diseases; the key may lie in how the immune response is capable of dealing with oral bacteria as well as with subsequent oral bacteremias. This could be comparable to a similar phenomenon observed in periodontal disease pathogenesis: as oral bacteria embedded in dental biofilms are necessary to challenge the host, the bacteria alone are not sufficient to cause disease (i.e., it takes a susceptible host to develop periodontal disease). For example, some patients with poor (or completely lack of) oral hygiene do not necessarily develop periodontal destruction; this is the result of a landmark cohort study that evaluated the natural history of periodontal disease occurrence in 480 Sri Lanka male patients with no access to oral care treatment or adequate oral hygiene practices. It found that 11% of patients showed no progression of periodontal disease beyond gingivitis [44]. Still, 8-13% of adults in the U.S. and Europe do develop moderate to severe generalized periodontitis that is less responsive to conventional periodontal therapy and have excellent access to oral care [45, 46]. These severe periodontitis patients ultimately experience tooth/bone loss and continued elevated systemic inflammation that could contribute to other chronic diseases [47]. Susceptibility to oral bacteremias, therefore, may follow a similar pattern in which the systemic response to oral bacteremias could be significantly detrimental in more susceptible patients.

Systemic Interactions of Oral Bacteremia and Its Potential Pathogenic Implications

Table 1 depicts relevant examples of bacterial genus (and species) of oral origin found in the blood and/or other body compartments. The "bacteremia route" is thought to start in the MALT-associated lymph vessels, trapping bacteria from the mouth to the bloodstream and then carry them to the vein of the venous angle near the supraclavicular area [48]. Once in circulation, oral bacteria can invade a wide array of body cells including immune cells where they evade immuno-surveillance and destruction. Some oral bacteria can also enter blood dendritic cells (DCs) or aggregate platelets to use them as "carriage". Eventually, oral bacteria reach different body compartments but the exact pathogenic role of this remote colonization is not quite clear. Oral bacteria are usually found and/or identified by means of molecular biology technology based on DNA or rRNA conserved gene sequences. Such techniques commonly require "DNA amplification" due to the low concentration of oral bacterial signatures, which suggests that the microbial load in remote sites tends to be significantly lower when compared to the bacterial load in the mouth. Nonetheless, some researchers have also reported cultivable viable oral bacteria from the blood or other body compartments, which supports the theory of immune evasion and bacterial survival to some extent. The following sections will discuss relevant scientific evidence of oral bacteria presence in the blood as well as in different systemic compartments in humans, as well as *in vitro* (Table 2) and *in vivo* (Table 3) experimental evidence that could explain in part the potential pathogenic consequences of oral bacteremia.

Oral Bacteria Presence in the Blood

Oral bacteremias have frequently been demonstrated in patients suffering from chronic periodontitis, particularly when these patients are treated with manual or ultrasonic scaling/root planing. [49-51]. Periodontal pathogens can be recovered from peripheral blood by means of haemoculture using specific enriched media and anaerobic culture conditions. However, such microbiology techniques offer limited sensitivity, as they usually require a threshold number of bacteria to demonstrate colony forming unit formations in the culture media [52]. Virulence factors from periodontal bacteria such as lipopolysaccharides have also been reported in the peripheral blood of periodontitis patients (i.e., endotoxemia) after gentle mastication, even more frequently in advanced severe cases [53, 54]. Indirect evidence of oral bacteremias has also been measured by assessing specific antibody titers against periodontal pathogens [55]. *Porphyromonas gingivalis* is uniquely able to invade/infect myeloid dendritic cells (mDCs) and this is more frequently observed in chronic periodontitis patients, especially when local debridement of the oral biofilm takes place [56].

Patients with a diseased periodontium can be a major (and underestimated) source of chronic and frequent release of bacterial pro-inflammatory components into the bloodstream in humans [53]. In fact, chronic periodontitis patients show significant elevations in circulating tumor necrosis factor (TNF-α) and interleukin (IL-6) after undergoing periodontal treatment [54]. TNF-α and IL-6 are known potent inducers of systemic inflammation, occasionally evidenced by pyrexia (fever) development following conventional periodontal treatment. The transitory but significant bacteremia could result in immune system stress with potential long-term deleterious effects in susceptible patients.

Oral bacteria can induce significant changes in blood cell behaviors. For example, *S. mutans* and *P. gingivalis* can induce platelet aggregation and increased adhesion molecules expression (e.g. P-selectin) *in vitro* [57, 58].

This is thought to make platelets more sluggish and stickier, contributing to plaque formation. *P. gingivalis* can also induce significant changes in DC functions; for example, different minor/major fimbriated *Pg* strains can dampen DCs maturation status and produce distinct immunomodulatory roles characterized by inflammatory cytokine profiles that result in either Th1 or Th2 effector responses [59, 60]. A non-canonical dendritic cell differentiation process can also be observed after *in vitro P .gingivalis* infection that influences immune homeostasis and promotes chronic inflammation [61]. Oral bacteria can also be detrimental to other immune cells such as lymphocytes and T cells; the effects range from Th1/Th2 activation [62] to CD4/CD8 cleavage and apoptosis induction [63-65], (Table 2).

Table 2. Pathogenic detrimental effects on different human cells after *in vitro* infection with oral bacteria*

Body system	Cell Type and Microorganism(s)	Effect(s)	References
Cardiovascular	Endothelial cells/*Streptococci*	Increased pro-inflammatory cytokine production, invasion	[80, 81]
	Endothelial cells/*P. gingivalis*	Enhanced inflammatory/coagulant responses	[207]
	Endothelial cells/*A. actinomycetemcomitans*	Pro-inflammatory effects, decreased proliferation	[208]
	Platelets/*S. mutans*	Aggregation induction	[57]
	Platelets/*P. gingivalis*	Increased P-selectin expression	[58]
Oral	Oral epithelial cells/*F. nucleatum*	Increased adhesion, invasion and IL-8 production	[111]
	Oral epithelial cells/*P. gingivalis* or *A. actinomycetemcomitans*	Invasion, focal adhesion degradation, enhanced proliferation, altered apoptosis	[209-212]
Immune	Lymphocytes/*F. nucleatum*	Apoptosis induction, T cell activation inhibition	[63, 64]
	T cells/*P. gingivalis*	CD4/CD8 cleavage by gingipains, Th1 or Th2 activation	[62, 65]
	Dendritic cells/*P. gingivalis*	Altered maturation, chemokine receptor profile reprogramming, homing disruption, increased migration towards inflammatory vascular sites, non-canonical differentiation, apoptosis resistance	[60, 61, 213]
Fetoplacental unit	Trophoblasts/*C. rectus*	Increased pro-inflammatory cytokine production, invasion	[110]
	Trophoblasts/P. gingivalis	Cell cycle arrest and apoptosis.	[112]

*Relevant literature examples have been included for illustration purposes, however several references were unintentionally excluded due to space limitations.

The use of antibiotics has been recommended to reduce the risk after oral bacteremia complications. There is some clinical evidence of the efficacy of Amoxicillin and Azithromycin in the prevention of bacteremia following dental procedures [66]. Oral rinses show less effectiveness in reducing bacteremia [67]. It is generally believed that although antibiotics do have an impact in reducing bacteremia, they do not completely eliminate bacteremia altogether [68]. New randomized clinical trials are currently taking place, which will offer a better understanding of the systemic effects of oral antibiotics in conjunction with conventional periodontal therapy in chronic periodontitis patients (ClinicalTrials.gov Identifier NCT01568944).

Oral Bacteria Presence in Cardiovascular Tissues

Cardiovascular tissues are probably the most studied human tissues in association to oral infections, and the associated oral bacteria have been linked to cardiovascular interactions in the last two decades. The presence of oral bacterial DNA has been frequently detected in carotid arterial plaques, coronary atheromatous vessel plaques, abdominal aortic aneurysmal walls, intraluminal thrombi aspirates, occluded arteries, phlebitis samples and primary varicose veins (frequency ranging from ~48-88%) [28, 48, 69-71]. Most epidemiological studies have proposed periodontal disease as an independent risk factor for cardiovascular diseases, however these associations are generally weaker when compared to other common risk factors such as smoking and history of other past infections [72]. The issue still remains highly controversial in both medical and dental communities [73-74].

There is however a considerable amount of evidence to support a biological plausibility between periodontitis and cardiovascular events. Cardiovascular diseases (CVD) are originated from repeated vascular endothelium injury and chronic inflammation [75], and oral infections are believed to contribute to both. For instance, in fulfillment of the modified Koch's postulates [76], a recent systematic review demonstrated substantial evidence for: 1) dissemination from the oral cavity to vascular tissues (Table 1); 2) oral bacteria can be found in affected tissues [77]; 3) Oral bacteria can live within affected sites [78, 79]; 4) Oral bacteria can invade vascular cell types (e.g. endothelial cells), induce inflammation and interact with platelets *in vitro* (Table 2), [80-82]; 5) Oral bacteria can induce atherosclerosis in animal models of disease (Table 3), [83-85] and 6) non-invasive mutants of oral bacteria cause significantly reduced pathology in animal models [84]. The last postulate to demonstrate human clinical isolates to cause disease in animal models has not been reported yet [86].

Table 3. Experimental animal models demonstrating systemic effects after induced bacteremia with oral pathogens*

Animal Model	System	Oral Microorganism(s) and infection route	Effect(s)	References
Mice	Cardiovascular	*P. gingivalis* via oral infection or IV injection	Cytokinemia, Atherosclerosis acceleration, endothelial progenitors mobilization	[84, 214-217]
		P. gingivalis via subcutaneous chamber	Autoimmune myocarditis induction	[218]
	GI tract	*S. mutans* via IV	Ulcerative colitis aggravation	[219]
	Fetoplacental Unit	*F. nucleatum* via IV	Premature and term stillbirths	[113]
		C. rectus via oral infection or subcutaneous chamber	Fetal growth restriction, placentitis, altered fecundity	[109, 110, 220]
	Joints/RA	Oral gavage with *P. gingivalis*	Faster and more severe arthritis development	[145]
Rat	Cardiovascular	*S. mutans* via IV	Infective endocarditis (IE)	[221]
	Fetoplacental Unit	P. gingivalis (or LPS) via IV infusion	Increased maternal blood pressure, fetal growth restriction/resorptions, chorioamnionitis/placentitis	[222, 223]
	Joints/RA	Subdermal heat-killed *P. gingivalis* injections	Paw swelling, Arthritis	[144]
Rabbit	Cardiovascular	*S. sanguis* via IV infusion P. gingivalis via IV injection	Platelets/fibrin aggregation Intimal thickening	[224,, 225]
	Fetoplacental Unit	*P. gingivalis* via subcutaneous chamber	Fetal translocation and exposure	[226]
Guinea pig	Cardiovascular	P. gingivalis proteinases via intradermal injections	Vascular permeability enhancement	[227]
Pig	Cardiovascular	*P. gingivalis* via IV injection	Coronary/aortic atherosclerosis	[85]
Sheep	Fetoplacental Unit	Pg, Aa, or Fn (LPS)	Higher fetal lethality rates when compared to E. coli	[228]
Non-human primate	Fetoplacental Unit	Induced periodontitis with ligatures	Increased inflammatory mediators, Cytokinemia, increased CRP (acute phase) protein induction	[119-231]

*Relevant literature examples have been included for illustration purposes, however several references were unintentionally excluded due to space limitations.

Other than oral bacterial invasion to affected cardiovascular tissues, indirect mechanisms promoting systemic inflammation in response to oral bacteria have also been proposed to have a role in the pathogenesis of CVD. Increased circulating inflammatory mediators present in periodontal disease patients can promote endothelial activation and atherogenesis. For example, C-reactive protein (CRP) is an acute-phase protein that is associated with future cardiovascular events and is frequently regarded as a biomarker of systemic inflammation [87]. Notably, patients with periodontal disease have significantly higher serum levels of several inflammatory mediators (fibrinogen, TNF-α, IL-1, IL-6) including C-reactive protein when compared to healthy controls [88, 89].

Cardiovascular function can also be indirectly assessed by means of non-invasive procedures to evaluate the blood vessel function as a surrogate marker for early cardiovascular disease. Endothelial dysfunction is a pathological stage of the endothelium characterized by an imbalance in dilation/contraction responses; flow-mediated, endothelium dependent vasodilatation of the brachial artery (FMD) evaluates endothelial function by means of controlled handcuff pressure on the brachial artery measured by ultrasound imaging [90, 91]. Interestingly, single-arm clinical trials have reported FMD improvement and reduction of systemic markers of inflammation after periodontal treatment in patients with severe periodontitis [92-94]. These observations strongly suggest that reducing periodontitis-associated bacteremia by means of periodontal treatment may be beneficial long term in some patients.

Oral Bacteria Presence in the Fetoplacental Unit

Periodontal disease and associated periodontopathogens have also been significantly associated with pregnancy complications including preterm delivery, low birth weight and preeclampsia [96-97]. In fact, important periodontal pathogens have been detected in human placentas of women with preterm delivery [98], preeclampsia [99] and in the amniotic fluid of pregnant women with a diagnosis of premature labor [100] or premature labor with intact membranes [101-106] and (Table 1). Fetal exposure to periodontal pathogens from maternal oral biofilms has also been demonstrated in umbilical cord blood samples from preterm births. Fetal immunoglobulin M (IgM) reacts to one or more specific oral pathogens such as *P. gingivalis* and *Campylobacter rectus*, suggesting an adaptive immune responses developed by the fetus against oral bacteremia from the mother [107, 108].

Placental infection and subsequent inflammation have been associated with the pathogenesis of most pregnancy complications. *In vitro* evidence suggests that placental cells (e.g. trophoblasts) do develop pro-inflammatory responses when exposed to and invaded by the oral pathogens *F. nucleatum* and *C. rectus* [109-111]. Placental cells can also undergo abnormal cell cycles and induced pathogenic apoptosis when exposed to *P. gingivalis* [112], (Table 2). Moreover, evidence derived from *in vivo* animal experiments is highly supportive of the oral bacteria/placental inflammation link; for example, IV injections of *F. nucleatum* induce placental inflammation and increased fetal resorptions and stillbirths in mice [113]. Systemic dissemination of periodontal pathogens in mice (*P. gingivalis* and *C. rectus*) has been shown in blood, liver, uteri and murine placentas of growth-restricted fetuses [114-116]. Fetal growth restriction and histological evidence of placental inflammation with areas of focal necrosis can be seen in orally infected mice [109], (Table 3).

The association between adverse pregnancy outcomes (APOs) and oral infections in humans is subject to scientific debate and controversy [97]. Recent large multicenter randomized clinical trials evaluating the effects of periodontal treatment have failed to prove a significant reduction in preterm delivery cases [117, 118] while others report significant effects [119-121]. All clinical research findings support that a transitory bacteremia in pregnant women after conventional periodontal therapy is safe and not detrimental; however therapy aiming to reduce local/systemic infection and bacteremia during pregnancy does not appear to be sufficient to reduce adverse pregnancy outcomes. Nevertheless, it would appear as if pathogenic features associated with APO's could be developed during the early stages of pregnancy, therefore limiting the effects of conventional periodontal therapy after the first trimester [122]. Furthermore, a more preventive and personalized targeted therapy in future and current pregnant women could have a more predictive outcome when compared to the evaluated "one-treatment-fits-all" periodontal treatment approach [108].

Oral Bacteria Presence in the Gastro-Intestinal Tract

The microbiota of the gut has been proposed to have an important role in the progression of colorectal cancer (CRC) and irritable bowel syndrome (IBS), and since the mucosa-associated microbiome in the gastro-intestinal tract is not isolated from that of the microbiome in the mouth, researchers have looked for potential implications of oral bacteria in the GI tract [123]. Interestingly, epidemiological observations have linked tooth loss/poor oral hygiene with increased risk of gastric cancer in different human populations [124-126]. Oral bacteria phyla such as *Fusobacterium*, *Porphyromonadaceae*,

Streptococcus and *Bacteroides* have been identified in CRC and IBS lesions and/or biopsies [127, 128]. Also, selected oral bacterial DNA can be found in gastric precancerous biopsies [129, 130].

Helicobacter pylorus is a classically known infectious agent associated with gastric cancer, and it is thought that 18% of cancers worldwide can be attributed to *H. pylori* colonization. *C. rectus* on the other hand is a Gram-negative anaerobe and motile bacterium unique to the oral cavity. *C. rectus* is highly phylogenetically related to *H. pylori* and is associated with ulceration of the periodontal attachment apparatus [131]. *C. rectus* strains possess proteinaceous antigens, including heat shock proteins that share antigenicity with antigens of *H. pylori strains*, and a potential cross-reactive antigen has been related to the induction of immunopathological responses in both periodontal tissues and the stomach [132]. Similarly, a number of recent bacterial genomic studies have strongly linked *Fusobacterium* spp. in colorectal carcinomas and associated lymph node metastasis [133, 134]. *F. nucleatum* has been reported to be the most dominant phylotype identified in these type of lesions [135]. Research has not yet elucidated how oral *Fusobacterium* infections could cause colon cancer, or whether colonization is a consequence of colon cancer, or something in between, but there is a belief that intestinal lumen microbiota can be affected by oral bacteria and potentially influence CRC risk. As to the infectious route, little is known related to the role of bacteremia in the gut colonization or whether oral bacteria utilize an enteral pathway for GI colonization.

Oral Bacteria Presence in the Joints of Rheumatoid Arthritis or Other Autoimmune Conditions

Rheumatoid arthritis (RA) is a chronic inflammatory disease characterized by inflammatory infiltrate accumulation in the synovial membrane of major body joints, which ultimately leads to local tissue destruction and impaired function. Environmental, genetic and immunological risk factors have been linked to RA pathogenesis, but the exact etiology is currently unknown. Some studies suggest that infectious agents can act as trigger factors in a susceptible host; the potential microorganisms involved are mycoplasma, Epstein–Barr virus, cytomegalovirus, rubeola virus and periodontal bacteria [136]. Remarkably, both periodontitis and RA share very similar disease mechanisms: the host mounts an immune response mediated by neutrophils, monocytes and T and B lymphocytes in response to bacteria/virulence factors challenge. These host-pathogen interactions lead to the overproduction of tissue proteinases, pro-inflammatory cytokines and prostaglandins. These stimulate osteoclastic activity and ultimately lead to bone or cartilage erosion [137]. Clinically, there is a statistically significant association between periodontal disease and RA in humans. For example, antibodies against oral pathogens and oral bacteria DNA have been isolated from both the sera and synovial fluids of RA patients [138-142], (Table 1). Also, responses against the free form of bacterial DNA may have pathogenic effects during the autoimmune RA destruction, as bacterial DNA contains CpG motifs with strong immunostimulatory effects [143].

Animal models are also supportive of PD-RA association (Table 3). For instance, the subdermal injection of heat-killed *P. gingivalis* in rats with RA stimulates paw swelling and arthritic development [144]; mice with induced periodontitis developed more severe arthritis at a faster rate [145]. Taken together, these experimental results support that PD caused by bacterial infection can increase inflammation in distant synovial tissues *in vivo* [146].

Patients with degenerative RA usually end up requiring surgical placement of joint prostheses. Prosthetic joint infections are rare but well-recognized complications causing significant morbidity and mortality [147]. Similarly to IE, antibiotic prophylaxis has been recommended in the past for the prevention of joint prosthesis infections, under clinical guidelines developed and revised by the American Dental Association (ADA) and the American Academy of Orthopaedic Surgeons (AAOS) in 1997 and 2003 [148].

The AAOS even recommended in 2009 that all joint replacement patients should have antibiotic prophylaxis for any dental procedure creating bacteremia [149]. However, these recommendations generated controversy, as no high-level evidence-based data are currently available supporting a beneficial effect of prophylaxis in risk reduction [150, 151]. Moreover, most of the available evidence comes from small case reports depicting patients developing acute signs of hip prosthesis infections with oral bacteria after non-invasive dental cleanings without previous antibiotic prophylaxis [152, 153]. In the past decade, significant advances in the understanding of prosthetic joint infections have been made. Long-lived biofilm infections can remain dormant for years before creating a clinically recognized infection [154]. Therefore, the goal for the prevention of infected joint replacements should aim towards oral health optimization prior to surgical therapy [155].

Oral Bacteria Presence in Non-Oral Body Abscesses

Non-oral body abscesses associated with oral bacteria have been reported extensively in the literature from rare abnormal cases. In fact, some of these reports come from post-mortem cases with initial unknown etiology. For example, periodontal bacteria such as *Fusobacterium nucleatum*, *Treponema denticola*, *Prevotella intermedia* and *P. gingivalis* have been found in a fatal pyogenic liver abscess (PLA) case [156]. Brain abscesses have been frequently linked to *Aggregatibacter actinomycetemcomitans* infections in the literature [157-166]. Other GI tract-related complications such as appendicitis, intraperitoneal or perirectal abscesses have been reported to harbor oral bacteria [167-171]. The role of oral bacteria infections in non-oral body abscesses is currently unknown and scarce animal models have evaluated potential linked mechanisms [172].

Conclusion: Prevention of Oral Bacteremia: Is it Necessary?

Based upon a thorough review of the literature we conclude that bacteremias of oral origin occur often and can result of normal daily activities, as well as common dental procedures. These bacteremias are of low grade but are more common in patients with untreated dental diseases such as active caries and periodontal disease. The true pathophysiological significance of these observations is still unclear, but the fact that oral bacteria have been identified in multiple organ systems and are associated with more severe chronic diseases is somewhat troubling. In patients with chronic untreated dental disease, systemic exposure to these oral bacteremias occurs through decades of life, leading to an accumulation of inflammatory damage of which the scope has not yet been identified. However, long-term effects of oral bacteremias in other systems may be more detrimental in susceptible patients. As personalized medicine develops and becomes available to clinicians, new research should help in understanding patient's individual risk to reduce the odds of experiencing severe oral diseases as well as other related systemic diseases. In the meantime, education/prevention and early dental interventions seem to be the best immediate strategy to improve systemic outcomes in the majority of patients.

References

[1] Price WA. Dental infections and related degenerative diseases: Some structural and biochemical factors. *Journal of the American Medical Association*. 1925;84(4):254-61.

[2] Pallasch TJ, Wahl MJ. Focal infection: new age or ancient history? *Endodontic Topics*. 2003;4(1):32-45.

[3] Jacobsohn PH, Kantor ML, Pihlstrom BL. The X-ray in dentistry, and the legacy of C. Edmund Kells: a commentary on Kells CE. The X-ray in dental practice. J Natl Dent Assoc 1920;7(3):241-272. *J Am Dent Assoc*. 2013 Feb;144(2):138-42.

[4] Ramirez JH, Arce R, Contreras A. Why must physicians know about oral diseases? *Teach Learn Med*. 2010 Apr;22(2):148-55.

[5] Aas JA, Paster BJ, Stokes LN, Olsen I, Dewhirst FE. Defining the normal bacterial flora of the oral cavity. *J Clin Microbiol*. [Comparative Study Research Support, N.I.H., Extramural Research Support, Non-U.S. Gov't]. 2005 Nov;43(11):5721-32.

[6] Gibbons RJ. Bacterial adhesion to oral tissues: a model for infectious diseases. *J Dent Res*. [Research Support, U.S. Gov't, P.H.S. Review]. 1989 May;68(5):750-60.

[7] Aas JA, Griffen AL, Dardis SR, Lee AM, Olsen I, Dewhirst FE, et al. Bacteria of dental caries in primary and permanent teeth in children and young adults. *J Clin Microbiol*. [Research Support, N.I.H., Extramural Research Support, Non-U.S. Gov't]. 2008 Apr;46(4):1407-17.

[8] Kumar PS, Griffen AL, Barton JA, Paster BJ, Moeschberger ML, Leys EJ. New bacterial species associated with chronic periodontitis. *J Dent Res*. [Research Support, U.S. Gov't, P.H.S.]. 2003 May;82(5):338-44.

[9] Paster BJ, Boches SK, Galvin JL, Ericson RE, Lau CN, Levanos VA, et al. Bacterial diversity in human subgingival plaque. *J Bacteriol*. [Research Support, U.S. Gov't, P.H.S.]. 2001 Jun;183(12):3770-83.

[10] Socransky SS, Haffajee AD. Dental biofilms: difficult therapeutic targets. *Periodontol* 2000. [Research Support, U.S. Gov't, P.H.S. Review]. 2002;28:12-55.

[11] Dewhirst FE, Chen T, Izard J, Paster BJ, Tanner ACR, Yu WH, et al. The Human Oral Microbiome. *J Bacteriol*. 2010 Oct;192(19):5002-17.

[12] Wright CJ, Burns LH, Jack AA, Back CR, Dutton LC, Nobbs AH, et al. Microbial interactions in building of communities. *Mol Oral Microbiol*. 2013 Apr;28(2):83-101.

[13] Gibbons RJ, van Houte J. Selective bacterial adherence to oral epithelial surfaces and its role as an ecological determinant. *Infect Immun.* 1971 Apr;3(4):567-73.

[14] Russell RR. Changing concepts in caries microbiology. *Am J Dent.* [Review]. 2009 Oct;22(5):304-10.

[15] Teles R, Teles F, Frias-Lopez J, Paster B, Haffajee A. Lessons learned and unlearned in periodontal microbiology. *Periodontol* 2000. [Research Support, N.I.H., Extramural]. 2013 Jun;62(1):95-162.

[16] Kuboniwa M, Tribble GD, Hendrickson EL, Amano A, Lamont RJ, Hackett M. Insights into the virulence of oral biofilms: discoveries from proteomics. Expert Rev Proteomics. [Research Support, N.I.H., Extramural Research Support, Non-U.S. Gov't Review]. 2012 Jun;9(3):311-23.

[17] Socransky SS, Haffajee AD, Cugini MA, Smith C, Kent RL, Jr. Microbial complexes in subgingival plaque. *J Clin Periodontol.* [Research Support, U.S. Gov't, P.H.S.]. 1998 Feb;25(2):134-44.

[18] Armitage GC. Learned and unlearned concepts in periodontal diagnostics: a 50-year perspective. Periodontol 2000. 2013 Jun;62(1): 20-36.

[19] Baelum V, Lopez R. Periodontal disease epidemiology - learned and unlearned? *Periodontol* 2000. 2013 Jun;62(1):37-58.

[20] Hajishengallis G, Lamont RJ. Beyond the red complex and into more complexity: the polymicrobial synergy and dysbiosis (PSD) model of periodontal disease etiology. *Mol Oral Microbiol.* [Research Support, N.I.H., Extramural]. 2012 Dec;27(6):409-19.

[21] Darveau RP. Periodontitis: a polymicrobial disruption of host homeostasis. *Nat Rev Microbiol.* 2010 Jul;8(7):481-90.

[22] Hajishengallis G, Liang S, Payne MA, Hashim A, Jotwani R, Eskan MA, et al. Low-Abundance Biofilm Species Orchestrates Inflammatory Periodontal Disease through the Commensal Microbiota and Complement. *Cell Host Microbe.* 2011 Nov 17;10(5):497-506.

[23] Tlaskalova-Hogenova H, Stepankova R, Hudcovic T, Tuckova L, Cukrowska B, Lodinova-Zadnikova R, et al. Commensal bacteria (normal microflora), mucosal immunity and chronic inflammatory and autoimmune diseases. *Immunol Lett.* [Research Support, Non-U.S. Gov't Review]. 2004 May 15;93(2-3):97-108.

[24] Uematsu S, Akira S. Toll-like receptors and innate immunity. *J Mol Med-Jmm.* 2006 Sep;84(9):712-25.

[25] Bartold PM, Walsh LJ, Narayanan S. Molecular and cell biology of the gingiva. *Periodontol* 2000. 2000;24:28-55.

[26] Colombo AV, da Silva CM, Haffajee A, Colombo APV. Identification of intracellular oral species within human crevicular epithelial cells from subjects with chronic periodontitis by fluorescence in situ hybridization. *J Periodontal Res*. 2007 Jun;42(3):236-43.

[27] Ebersole JL, Dawson DR, 3rd, Morford LA, Peyyala R, Miller CS, Gonzalez OA. Periodontal disease immunology: 'double indemnity' in protecting the host. *Periodontol* 2000. 2013 Jun;62(1):163-202.

[28] Ford PJ, Gemmell E, Hamlet SM, Hasan A, Walker PJ, West MJ, et al. Cross-reactivity of GroEL antibodies with human heat shock protein 60 and quantification of pathogens in atherosclerosis. *Oral Microbiol Immunol.* [Comparative Study Research Support, Non-U.S. Gov't]. 2005 Oct;20(5):296-302.

[29] Figuero E, Sanchez-Beltran M, Cuesta-Frechoso S, Tejerina JM, del Castro JA, Gutierrez JM, et al. Detection of periodontal bacteria in atheromatous plaque by nested polymerase chain reaction. *J Periodontol.* 2011 Oct;82(10):1469-77.

[30] Crasta K, Daly CG, Mitchell D, Curtis B, Stewart D, Heitz-Mayfield LJ. Bacteraemia due to dental flossing. *J Clin Periodontol.* [Research Support, Non-U.S. Gov't]. 2009 Apr;36(4):323-32.

[31] Pallasch TJ. Antibiotic prophylaxis: problems in paradise. *Dent Clin North Am.* [Review]. 2003 Oct;47(4):665-79.

[32] Tomas I, Diz P, Tobias A, Scully C, Donos N. Periodontal health status and bacteraemia from daily oral activities: systematic review/meta-analysis. *J Clin Periodontol.* 2012 Mar;39(3):213-28.

[33] Lockhart PB, Brennan MT, Sasser HC, Fox PC, Paster BJ, Bahrani-Mougeot FK. Bacteremia associated with toothbrushing and dental extraction. *Circulation.* [Comparative Study Randomized Controlled Trial Research Support, N.I.H., Extramural]. 2008 Jun 17;117(24):3118-25.

[34] Lockhart PB, Brennan MT, Thornhill M, Michalowicz BS, Noll J, Bahrani-Mougeot FK, et al. Poor oral hygiene as a risk factor for infective endocarditis-related bacteremia. *J Am Dent Assoc.* [Randomized Controlled Trial Research Support, N.I.H., Extramural Research Support, Non-U.S. Gov't]. 2009 Oct;140(10):1238-44.

[35] Berlin JA, Abrutyn E, Strom BL, Kinman JL, Levison ME, Korzeniowski OM, et al. Incidence of infective endocarditis in the

Delaware Valley, 1988-1990. *Am J Cardiol.* [Research Support, U.S. Gov't, P.H.S.]. 1995 Nov 1;76(12):933-6.

[36] Thornhill MH. Infective endocarditis: the impact of the NICE guidelines for antibiotic prophylaxis. *Dent Update.* 2012 Jan-Feb;39(1):6-10, 2.

[37] PREVENTION of rheumatic fever and bacterial endocarditis through control of streptococcal infections. *Pediatrics.* 1955 May;15(5):642-6.

[38] Wilson W, Taubert KA, Gewitz M, Lockhart PB, Baddour LM, Levison M, et al. Prevention of infective endocarditis: guidelines from the American Heart Association: a guideline from the American Heart Association Rheumatic Fever, Endocarditis, and Kawasaki Disease Committee, Council on Cardiovascular Disease in the Young, and the Council on Clinical Cardiology, Council on Cardiovascular Surgery and Anesthesia, and the Quality of Care and Outcomes Research Interdisciplinary Working Group. *Circulation.* [Practice Guideline]. 2007 Oct 9;116(15):1736-54.

[39] Wilson W, Taubert KA, Gewitz M, Lockhart PB, Baddour LM, Levison M, et al. Prevention of infective endocarditis: guidelines from the American Heart Association: a guideline from the American Heart Association Rheumatic Fever, Endocarditis and Kawasaki Disease Committee, Council on Cardiovascular Disease in the Young, and the Council on Clinical Cardiology, Council on Cardiovascular Surgery and Anesthesia, and the Quality of Care and Outcomes Research Interdisciplinary Working Group. *J Am Dent Assoc.* [Practice Guideline Review]. 2008 Jan;139 Suppl:3S-24S.

[40] Sakamoto H, Karakida K, Otsuru M, Aoki T, Hata Y, Aki A. Antibiotic prevention of infective endocarditis due to oral procedures: myth, magic, or science? *J Infect Chemother.* [Review]. 2007 Aug;13(4):189-95.

[41] Thornhill MH, Dayer MJ, Forde JM, Corey GR, Chu VH, Couper DJ, et al. Impact of the NICE guideline recommending cessation of antibiotic prophylaxis for prevention of infective endocarditis: before and after study. *Bmj.* [Research Support, Non-U.S. Gov't]. 2011;342:d2392.

[42] Veloso TR, Amiguet M, Rousson V, Giddey M, Vouillamoz J, Moreillon P, et al. Induction of Experimental Endocarditis by Continuous Low-Grade Bacteremia Mimicking Spontaneous Bacteremia in Humans. *Infect Immun.* 2011 May;79(5):2006-11.

[43] Roberts GJ. Dentists are innocent! "Everyday" bacteremia is the real culprit: A review and assessment of the evidence that dental surgical procedures are a principal cause of bacterial endocarditis in children. *Pediatr Cardiol.* 1999 Sep-Oct;20(5):317-25.

[44] Loe H, Anerud A, Boysen H, Morrison E. Natural history of periodontal disease in man. Rapid, moderate and no loss of attachment in Sri Lankan laborers 14 to 46 years of age. *J Clin Periodontol.* 1986 May;13(5):431-45.

[45] Hirschfeld L, Wasserman B. A long-term survey of tooth loss in 600 treated periodontal patients. *J Periodontol.* [Comparative Study]. 1978 May;49(5):225-37.

[46] Lindhe J, Nyman S. Long-term maintenance of patients treated for advanced periodontal disease. *J Clin Periodontol.* [Research Support, U.S. Gov't, P.H.S.]. 1984 Sep;11(8):504-14.

[47] Kornman KS, Duff GW. Personalized medicine: will dentistry ride the wave or watch from the beach? *J Dent Res.* 2012 Jul;91(7 Suppl):8S-11S.

[48] Iwai T. Periodontal bacteremia and various vascular diseases. *J Periodontal Res.* [Review]. 2009 Dec;44(6):689-94.

[49] Forner L, Larsen T, Kilian M, Holmstrup P. Incidence of bacteremia after chewing, tooth brushing and scaling in individuals with periodontal inflammation. *J Clin Periodontol.* [Research Support, Non-U.S. Gov't]. 2006 Jun;33(6):401-7.

[50] Castillo DM, Sanchez-Beltran MC, Castellanos JE, Sanz I, Mayorga-Fayad I, Sanz M, et al. Detection of specific periodontal microorganisms from bacteraemia samples after periodontal therapy using molecular-based diagnostics. *J Clin Periodontol.* [Comparative Study Research Support, Non-U.S. Gov't]. 2011 May;38(5):418-27.

[51] Lafaurie GI, Mayorga-Fayad I, Torres MF, Castillo DM, Aya MR, Baron A, et al. Periodontopathic microorganisms in peripheric blood after scaling and root planing. *J Clin Periodontol.* [Research Support, Non-U.S. Gov't]. 2007 Oct;34(10):873-9.

[52] Messini M, Skourti I, Markopulos E, Koutsia-Carouzou C, Kyriakopoulou E, Kostaki S, et al. Bacteremia after dental treatment in mentally handicapped people. *J Clin Periodontol.* 1999 Jul;26(7):469-73.

[53] Geerts SO, Nys M, De MP, Charpentier J, Albert A, Legrand V, et al. Systemic release of endotoxins induced by gentle mastication: association with periodontitis severity. *J Periodontol.* [Research Support, Non-U.S. Gov't]. 2002 Jan;73(1):73-8.

[54] Ide M, Jagdev D, Coward PY, Crook M, Barclay GR, Wilson RF. The short-term effects of treatment of chronic periodontitis on circulating levels of endotoxin, C-reactive protein, tumor necrosis factor-alpha, and

interleukin-6. *J Periodontol.* [Research Support, Non-U.S. Gov't]. 2004 Mar;75(3):420-8.

[55] Mustapha IZ, Debrey S, Oladubu M, Ugarte R. Markers of systemic bacterial exposure in periodontal disease and cardiovascular disease risk: a systematic review and meta-analysis. *J Periodontol.* [Meta-Analysis Research Support, N.I.H., Extramural Review]. 2007 Dec;78(12):2289-302.

[56] Carrion J, Scisci E, Miles B, Sabino GJ, Zeituni AE, Gu Y, et al. Microbial carriage state of peripheral blood dendritic cells (DCs) in chronic periodontitis influences DC differentiation, atherogenic potential. *J Immunol.* [Research Support, N.I.H., Extramural]. 2012 Sep 15;189(6):3178-87.

[57] Chia JS, Lin YL, Lien HT, Chen JY. Platelet aggregation induced by serotype polysaccharides from Streptococcus mutans. *Infect Immun.* [*In vitro* Research Support, Non-U.S. Gov't]. 2004 May;72(5):2605-17.

[58] Assinger A, Buchberger E, Laky M, Esfandeyari A, Brostjan C, Volf I. Periodontopathogens induce soluble P-selectin release by endothelial cells and platelets. *Thromb Res.* [Research Support, Non-U.S. Gov't]. 2011 Jan;127(1):e20-6.

[59] Zeituni AE, Jotwani R, Carrion J, Cutler CW. Targeting of DC-SIGN on human dendritic cells by minor fimbriated Porphyromonas gingivalis strains elicits a distinct effector T cell response. *J Immunol.* [Research Support, N.I.H., Extramural Research Support, U.S. Gov't, P.H.S.]. 2009 Nov 1;183(9):5694-704.

[60] Zeituni AE, Carrion J, Cutler CW. Porphyromonas gingivalis-dendritic cell interactions: consequences for coronary artery disease. *J Oral Microbiol.* 2010;2.

[61] Miles B, Scisci E, Carrion J, Sabino GJ, Genco CA, Cutler CW. Noncanonical dendritic cell differentiation and survival driven by a bacteremic pathogen. *J Leukoc Biol.* 2013 Aug;94(2):281-9.

[62] Vernal R, Diaz-Guerra E, Silva A, Sanz M, Garcia-Sanz JA. Distinct human T-lymphocyte responses triggered by Porphyromonas gingivalis capsular serotypes. *J Clin Periodontol.* 2013 Oct 3.

[63] Kaplan CW, Lux R, Huynh T, Jewett A, Shi W, Haake SK. Fusobacterium nucleatum apoptosis-inducing outer membrane protein. *J Dent Res.* [Research Support, N.I.H., Extramural Research Support, Non-U.S. Gov't]. 2005 Aug;84(8):700-4.

[64] Shenker BJ, Datar S. Fusobacterium nucleatum inhibits human T-cell activation by arresting cells in the mid-G1 phase of the cell cycle. *Infect*

Immun. [Research Support, U.S. Gov't, P.H.S.]. 1995 Dec;63(12): 4830-6.
[65] Kitamura Y, Matono S, Aida Y, Hirofuji T, Maeda K. Gingipains in the culture supernatant of Porphyromonas gingivalis cleave CD4 and CD8 on human T cells. *J Periodontal Res.* [Research Support, Non-U.S. Gov't]. 2002 Dec;37(6):464-8.
[66] Tomas Carmona I, Diz Dios P, Scully C. Efficacy of antibiotic prophylactic regimens for the prevention of bacterial endocarditis of oral origin. *J Dent Res.* [Evaluation Studies Review]. 2007 Dec;86(12):1142-59.
[67] Morozumi T, Kubota T, Abe D, Shimizu T, Komatsu Y, Yoshie H. Effects of irrigation with an antiseptic and oral administration of azithromycin on bacteremia caused by scaling and root planing. *J Periodontol.* [Comparative Study Randomized Controlled Trial Research Support, Non-U.S. Gov't]. 2010 Nov;81(11):1555-63.
[68] Brennan MT, Kent ML, Fox PC, Norton HJ, Lockhart PB. The impact of oral disease and nonsurgical treatment on bacteremia in children. *J Am Dent Assoc.* [Comparative Study Randomized Controlled Trial]. 2007 Jan;138(1):80-5.
[69] Kurihara N, Inoue Y, Iwai T, Sugano N, Umeda M, Huang Y, et al. Oral bacteria are a possible risk factor for valvular incompetence in primary varicose veins. *Eur J Vasc Endovasc Surg*. 2007 Jul;34(1):102-6.
[70] Kurihara N, Inoue Y, Iwai T, Umeda M, Huang Y, Ishikawa I. Detection and localization of periodontopathic bacteria in abdominal aortic aneurysms. *Eur J Vasc Endovasc Surg*. 2004 Nov;28(5):553-8.
[71] Ford PJ, Gemmell E, Chan A, Carter CL, Walker PJ, Bird PS, et al. Inflammation, heat shock proteins and periodontal pathogens in atherosclerosis: an immunohistologic study. *Oral Microbiol Immunol.* [Research Support, Non-U.S. Gov't]. 2006 Aug;21(4):206-11.
[72] Tonetti MS, Van Dyke TE. Periodontitis and atherosclerotic cardiovascular disease: consensus report of the Joint EFP/AAP Workshop on Periodontitis and Systemic Diseases. *J Periodontol.* 2013 Apr;84(4 Suppl):S24-9.
[73] Lockhart PB, Bolger AF, Papapanou PN, Osinbowale O, Trevisan M, Levison ME, et al. Periodontal disease and atherosclerotic vascular disease: does the evidence support an independent association?: a scientific statement from the American Heart Association. *Circulation.* [Consensus Development Conference]. 2012 May 22;125(20):2520-44.

[74] Papapanou PN, Trevisan M. Periodontitis and atherosclerotic vascular disease: what we know and why it is important. *J Am Dent Assoc.* [Editorial]. 2012 Aug;143(8):826-8.

[75] Ross R. Atherosclerosis--an inflammatory disease. *N Engl J Med.* [Research Support, U.S. Gov't, P.H.S. Review]. 1999 Jan 14;340(2):115-26.

[76] Socransky SS. Criteria for the infectious agents in dental caries and periodontal disease. *J Clin Periodontol.* 1979 Dec;6(7):16-21.

[77] Haraszthy VI, Zambon JJ, Trevisan M, Zeid M, Genco RJ. Identification of periodontal pathogens in atheromatous plaques. *J Periodontol.* 2000 Oct;71(10):1554-60.

[78] Kozarov EV, Dorn BR, Shelburne CE, Dunn WA, Jr., Progulske-Fox A. Human atherosclerotic plaque contains viable invasive Actinobacillus actinomycetemcomitans and Porphyromonas gingivalis. *Arterioscler Thromb Vasc Biol.* [Letter Research Support, N.I.H., Extramural Research Support, Non-U.S. Gov't Research Support, U.S. Gov't, P.H.S.]. 2005 Mar;25(3):e17-8.

[79] Rafferty B, Jonsson D, Kalachikov S, Demmer RT, Nowygrod R, Elkind MS, et al. Impact of monocytic cells on recovery of uncultivable bacteria from atherosclerotic lesions. *J Intern Med.* [Research Support, N.I.H., Extramural Research Support, Non-U.S. Gov't]. 2011 Sep;270(3):273-80.

[80] de Toledo A, Nagata E, Yoshida Y, Oho T. Streptococcus oralis coaggregation receptor polysaccharides induce inflammatory responses in human aortic endothelial cells. *Mol Oral Microbiol.* [Research Support, Non-U.S. Gov't]. 2012 Aug;27(4):295-307.

[81] Nagata E, de Toledo A, Oho T. Invasion of human aortic endothelial cells by oral viridans group streptococci and induction of inflammatory cytokine production. *Mol Oral Microbiol.* [Comparative Study Research Support, Non-U.S. Gov't]. 2011 Feb;26(1):78-88.

[82] Fitzgerald JR, Foster TJ, Cox D. The interaction of bacterial pathogens with platelets. *Nature reviews Microbiology.* [Research Support, Non-U.S. Gov't Review]. 2006 Jun;4(6):445-57.

[83] Lalla E, Lamster IB, Hofmann MA, Bucciarelli L, Jerud AP, Tucker S, et al. Oral infection with a periodontal pathogen accelerates early atherosclerosis in apolipoprotein E-null mice. *Arterioscler Thromb Vasc Biol.* [Research Support, Non-U.S. Gov't Research Support, U.S. Gov't, P.H.S.]. 2003 Aug 1;23(8):1405-11.

[84] Gibson FC, 3rd, Hong C, Chou HH, Yumoto H, Chen J, Lien E, et al. Innate immune recognition of invasive bacteria accelerates atherosclerosis in apolipoprotein E-deficient mice. *Circulation.* [Research Support, U.S. Gov't, P.H.S.]. 2004 Jun 8;109(22):2801-6.

[85] Brodala N, Merricks EP, Bellinger DA, Damrongsri D, Offenbacher S, Beck J, et al. Porphyromonas gingivalis bacteremia induces coronary and aortic atherosclerosis in normocholesterolemic and hypercholesterolemic pigs. *Arterioscler Thromb Vasc Biol.* [Research Support, N.I.H., Extramural Research Support, U.S. Gov't, P.H.S.]. 2005 Jul;25(7):1446-51.

[86] Reyes L, Herrera D, Kozarov E, Rolda S, Progulske-Fox A. Periodontal bacterial invasion and infection: contribution to atherosclerotic pathology. *J Periodontol.* 2013 Apr;84(4 Suppl):S30-50.

[87] Ridker PM. Clinical application of C-reactive protein for cardiovascular disease detection and prevention. *Circulation.* [Research Support, Non-U.S. Gov't Research Support, U.S. Gov't, P.H.S. Review]. 2003 Jan 28;107(3):363-9.

[88] Paraskevas S, Huizinga JD, Loos BG. A systematic review and meta-analyses on C-reactive protein in relation to periodontitis. *J Clin Periodontol.* [Meta-Analysis Research Support, Non-U.S. Gov't Review]. 2008 Apr;35(4):277-90.

[89] Joshipura KJ, Wand HC, Merchant AT, Rimm EB. Periodontal disease and biomarkers related to cardiovascular disease. *J Dent Res.* [Research Support, U.S. Gov't, P.H.S.]. 2004 Feb;83(2):151-5.

[90] Celermajer DS, Sorensen KE, Gooch VM, Spiegelhalter DJ, Miller OI, Sullivan ID, et al. Non-invasive detection of endothelial dysfunction in children and adults at risk of atherosclerosis. *Lancet.* [Research Support, Non-U.S. Gov't]. 1992 Nov 7;340(8828):1111-5.

[91] Ramirez JH, Arce RM, Contreras A. Periodontal treatment effects on endothelial function and cardiovascular disease biomarkers in subjects with chronic periodontitis: protocol for a randomized clinical trial. *Trials.* 2011;12:46.

[92] Elter JR, Hinderliter AL, Offenbacher S, Beck JD, Caughey M, Brodala N, et al. The effects of periodontal therapy on vascular endothelial function: a pilot trial. *Am Heart J.* [Research Support, N.I.H., Extramural]. 2006 Jan;151(1):47.

[93] Mercanoglu F, Oflaz H, Oz O, Gokbuget AY, Genchellac H, Sezer M, et al. Endothelial dysfunction in patients with chronic periodontitis and its

improvement after initial periodontal therapy. *J Periodontol.* 2004 Dec;75(12):1694-700.
[94] Tonetti MS, D'Aiuto F, Nibali L, Donald A, Storry C, Parkar M, et al. Treatment of periodontitis and endothelial function. *N Engl J Med.* [Randomized Controlled Trial Research Support, Non-U.S. Gov't]. 2007 Mar 1;356(9):911-20.
[95] Offenbacher S, Boggess KA, Murtha AP, Jared HL, Lieff S, McKaig RG, et al. Progressive periodontal disease and risk of very preterm delivery. *ObstetGynecol.* 2006;107(1):29-36.
[96] Contreras A, Herrera JA, Soto JE, Arce RM, Jaramillo A, Botero JE. Periodontitis is associated with preeclampsia in pregnant women. *J Periodontol.* 2006 Feb;77(2):182-8.
[97] Ide M, Papapanou PN. Epidemiology of association between maternal periodontal disease and adverse pregnancy outcomes--systematic review. *J Periodontol.* 2013 Apr;84(4 Suppl):S181-94.
[98] Katz J, Chegini N, Shiverick KT, Lamont RJ. Localization of P. gingivalis in preterm delivery placenta. *J Dent Res.* [Research Support, N.I.H., Extramural Research Support, Non-U.S. Gov't]. 2009 Jun;88(6):575-8.
[99] Barak S, Oettinger-Barak O, Machtei EE, Sprecher H, Ohel G. Evidence of periopathogenic microorganisms in placentas of women with preeclampsia. *J Periodontol.* [Research Support, Non-U.S. Gov't]. 2007 Apr;78(4):670-6.
[100] Leon R, Silva N, Ovalle A, Chaparro A, Ahumada A, Gajardo M, et al. Detection of Porphyromonas gingivalis in the amniotic fluid in pregnant women with a diagnosis of threatened premature labor. *J Periodontol.* [Research Support, Non-U.S. Gov't]. 2007 Jul;78(7):1249-55.
[101] Chaim W, Mazor M. Intraamniotic infection with fusobacteria. *ArchGynecolObstet.* 1992;251(1):1-7.
[102] Gardella C, Riley DE, Hitti J, Agnew K, Krieger JN, Eschenbach D. Identification and sequencing of bacterial rDNAs in culture-negative amniotic fluid from women in premature labor. *AmJPerinatol.* 2004;21(6):319-23.
[103] Bohrer JC, Kamemoto LE, Almeida PG, Ogasawara KK. Acute chorioamnionitis at term caused by the oral pathogen Fusobacterium nucleatum. *Hawaii J Med Public Health.* [Case Reports]. 2012 Oct;71(10):280-1.

[104] Dixon NG, Ebright D, Defrancesco MA, Hawkins RE. Orogenital contact: a cause of chorioamnionitis? *Obstet Gynecol.* [Case Reports]. 1994 Oct;84(4 Pt 2):654-5.

[105] Garnier F, Masson G, Bedu A, Masson P, Decroisette E, Guigonis V, et al. Maternofetal infections due to Eikenella corrodens. *J Med Microbiol.* [Case Reports]. 2009 Feb;58(Pt 2):273-5.

[106] Han YW. Oral Health and Adverse Pregnancy Outcomes - What's Next? *JDentRes.* 2011;90(3):289-93.

[107] Madianos PN, Lieff S, Murtha AP, Boggess KA, Auten RL, Jr., Beck JD, et al. Maternal periodontitis and prematurity. Part II: Maternal infection and fetal exposure. *Ann Periodontol.* [Comparative Study Research Support, U.S. Gov't, P.H.S.]. 2001 Dec;6(1):175-82.

[108] Madianos PN, Bobetsis YA, Offenbacher S. Adverse pregnancy outcomes (APOs) and periodontal disease: pathogenic mechanisms. *J Periodontol.* 2013 Apr;84(4 Suppl):S170-80.

[109] Arce RM, Barros SP, Wacker B, Peters B, Moss K, Offenbacher S. Increased TLR4 expression in murine placentas after oral infection with periodontal pathogens. *Placenta.* 2009 Feb;30(2):156-62.

[110] Arce RM, Diaz PI, Barros SP, Galloway P, Bobetsis Y, Threadgill D, et al. Characterization of the invasive and inflammatory traits of oral Campylobacter rectus in a murine model of fetoplacental growth restriction and in trophoblast cultures. *J Reprod Immunol.* 2010 Mar;84(2):145-53.

[111] Han YW, Shi W, Huang GT, Kinder Haake S, Park NH, Kuramitsu H, et al. Interactions between periodontal bacteria and human oral epithelial cells: Fusobacterium nucleatum adheres to and invades epithelial cells. *Infect Immun.* [Research Support, U.S. Gov't, P.H.S.]. 2000 Jun;68(6):3140-6.

[112] Inaba H, Kuboniwa M, Bainbridge B, Yilmaz O, Katz J, Shiverick KT, et al. Porphyromonas gingivalis invades human trophoblasts and inhibits proliferation by inducing G1 arrest and apoptosis. *Cell Microbiol.* [Research Support, N.I.H., Extramural]. 2009 Oct;11(10):1517-32.

[113] Han YW, Redline RW, Li M, Yin L, Hill GB, McCormick TS. Fusobacterium nucleatum induces premature and term stillbirths in pregnant mice: implication of oral bacteria in preterm birth. *Infect Immun.* [Research Support, Non-U.S. Gov't Research Support, U.S. Gov't, P.H.S.]. 2004 Apr;72(4):2272-9.

[114] Lin D, Smith MA, Elter J, Champagne C, Downey CL, Beck J, et al. Porphyromonas gingivalis infection in pregnant mice is associated with

placental dissemination, an increase in the placental Th1/Th2 cytokine ratio, and fetal growth restriction. *InfectImmun.* 2003;71(9):5163-8.

[115] Offenbacher S, Riche EL, Barros SP, Bobetsis YA, Lin D, Beck JD. Effects of maternal Campylobacter rectus infection on murine placenta, fetal and neonatal survival, and brain development. *JPeriodontol.* 2005;76(11 Suppl):2133-43.

[116] Yeo A, Smith MA, Lin D, Riche EL, Moore A, Elter J, et al. Campylobacter rectus mediates growth restriction in pregnant mice. *JPeriodontol.* 2005;76(4):551-7.

[117] Offenbacher S, Beck JD, Jared HL, Mauriello SM, Mendoza LC, Couper DJ, et al. Effects of periodontal therapy on rate of preterm delivery: a randomized controlled trial. *ObstetGynecol.* 2009;114(3):551-9.

[118] Michalowicz BS, Gustafsson A, Thumbigere-Math V, Buhlin K. The effects of periodontal treatment on pregnancy outcomes. *J Periodontol.* 2013 Apr;84(4 Suppl):S195-208.

[119] Lopez NJ, Smith PC, Gutierrez J. Higher risk of preterm birth and low birth weight in women with periodontal disease. *JDentRes.* 2002;81(1):58-63.

[120] Chambrone L, Pannuti CM, Guglielmetti MR, Chambrone LA. Evidence grade associating periodontitis with preterm birth and/or low birth weight: II: a systematic review of randomized trials evaluating the effects of periodontal treatment. *J Clin Periodontol.* [Meta-Analysis Review]. 2011 Oct;38(10):902-14.

[121] Gazolla CM, Ribeiro A, Moyses MR, Oliveira LA, Pereira LJ, Sallum AW. Evaluation of the incidence of preterm low birth weight in patients undergoing periodontal therapy. *J Periodontol.* [Controlled Clinical Trial]. 2007 May;78(5):842-8.

[122] Offenbacher S, Beck J. Has periodontal treatment failed to reduce adverse pregnancy outcomes? The answer may be premature. *JPeriodontol.* 2007;78(2):195-7.

[123] Nell S, Suerbaum S, Josenhans C. The impact of the microbiota on the pathogenesis of IBD: lessons from mouse infection models. *Nature reviews Microbiology.* [Research Support, Non-U.S. Gov't Review]. 2010 Aug;8(8):564-77.

[124] Abnet CC, Kamangar F, Dawsey SM, Stolzenberg-Solomon RZ, Albanes D, Pietinen P, et al. Tooth loss is associated with increased risk of gastric non-cardia adenocarcinoma in a cohort of Finnish smokers. *Scand J Gastroenterol.* [Comparative Study Research Support, N.I.H.,

Extramural Research Support, U.S. Gov't, P.H.S.]. 2005 Jun;40(6): 681-7.

[125] Abnet CC, Qiao YL, Mark SD, Dong ZW, Taylor PR, Dawsey SM. Prospective study of tooth loss and incident esophageal and gastric cancers in China. *Cancer Causes Control.* 2001 Nov;12(9):847-54.

[126] Michaud DS, Liu Y, Meyer M, Giovannucci E, Joshipura K. Periodontal disease, tooth loss, and cancer risk in male health professionals: a prospective cohort study. *Lancet Oncol.* [Research Support, N.I.H., Extramural]. 2008 Jun;9(6):550-8.

[127] Chen W, Liu F, Ling Z, Tong X, Xiang C. Human intestinal lumen and mucosa-associated microbiota in patients with colorectal cancer. *Plos One.* [Research Support, Non-U.S. Gov't]. 2012;7(6):e39743.

[128] Rigsbee L, Agans R, Shankar V, Kenche H, Khamis HJ, Michail S, et al. Quantitative profiling of gut microbiota of children with diarrhea-predominant irritable bowel syndrome. *Am J Gastroenterol.* [Research Support, N.I.H., Extramural]. 2012 Nov;107(11):1740-51.

[129] Salazar CR, Francois F, Li Y, Corby P, Hays R, Leung C, et al. Association between oral health and gastric precancerous lesions. *Carcinogenesis.* [Research Support, N.I.H., Extramural]. 2012 Feb;33(2):399-403.

[130] Salazar CR, Sun J, Li Y, Francois F, Corby P, Perez-Perez G, et al. Association between selected oral pathogens and gastric precancerous lesions. *Plos One.* [Research Support, N.I.H., Extramural]. 2013;8(1):e51604.

[131] Rams TE, Feik D, Slots J. Campylobacter rectus in human periodontitis. *Oral MicrobiolImmunol.* 1993;8(4):230-5.

[132] Okuda K, Kimizuka R, Katakura A, Nakagawa T, Ishihara K. Ecological and immunopathological implications of oral bacteria in Helicobacter pylori-infected disease. *J Periodontol.* [Research Support, Non-U.S. Gov't Review]. 2003 Jan;74(1):123-8.

[133] Castellarin M, Warren RL, Freeman JD, Dreolini L, Krzywinski M, Strauss J, et al. Fusobacterium nucleatum infection is prevalent in human colorectal carcinoma. *Genome Res.* [Research Support, Non-U.S. Gov't]. 2012 Feb;22(2):299-306.

[134] Kostic AD, Gevers D, Pedamallu CS, Michaud M, Duke F, Earl AM, et al. Genomic analysis identifies association of Fusobacterium with colorectal carcinoma. *Genome Res.* [Research Support, N.I.H., Extramural Research Support, Non-U.S. Gov't]. 2012 Feb;22(2):292-8.

[135] Ray K. Colorectal cancer: Fusobacterium nucleatum found in colon cancer tissue--could an infection cause colorectal cancer? *Nat Rev Gastroenterol Hepatol.* [Comment]. 2011 Dec;8(12):662.

[136] Bartold PM, Marshall RI, Haynes DR. Periodontitis and rheumatoid arthritis: a review. *J Periodontol.* [Review]. 2005 Nov;76(11 Suppl):2066-74.

[137] Mercado FB, Marshall RI, Klestov AC, Bartold PM. Relationship between rheumatoid arthritis and periodontitis. *J Periodontol.* [Comparative Study Research Support, Non-U.S. Gov't]. 2001 Jun;72(6):779-87.

[138] Ogrendik M. Does periodontopathic bacterial infection contribute to the etiopathogenesis of the autoimmune disease rheumatoid arthritis? *Discov Med.* 2012 May;13(72):349-55.

[139] Moen K, Brun JG, Valen M, Skartveit L, Eribe EK, Olsen I, et al. Synovial inflammation in active rheumatoid arthritis and psoriatic arthritis facilitates trapping of a variety of oral bacterial DNAs. *Clin Exp Rheumatol.* [Research Support, Non-U.S. Gov't]. 2006 Nov-Dec;24(6):656-63.

[140] Ogrendik M, Kokino S, Ozdemir F, Bird PS, Hamlet S. Serum antibodies to oral anaerobic bacteria in patients with rheumatoid arthritis. *MedGenMed.* [Clinical Trial Multicenter Study]. 2005;7(2):2.

[141] Cox CJ, Kempsell KE, Gaston JS. Investigation of infectious agents associated with arthritis by reverse transcription PCR of bacterial rRNA. *Arthritis Res Ther.* [Research Support, Non-U.S. Gov't]. 2003;5(1):R1-8.

[142] Sun W, Dong L, Kaneyama K, Takegami T, Segami N. Bacterial diversity in synovial fluids of patients with TMD determined by cloning and sequencing analysis of the 16S ribosomal RNA gene. *Oral Surg Oral Med Oral Pathol Oral Radiol Endod.* [Research Support, Non-U.S. Gov't]. 2008 May;105(5):566-71.

[143] Martinez-Martinez RE, Abud-Mendoza C, Patino-Marin N, Rizo-Rodriguez JC, Little JW, Loyola-Rodriguez JP. Detection of periodontal bacterial DNA in serum and synovial fluid in refractory rheumatoid arthritis patients. *J Clin Periodontol.* [Research Support, Non-U.S. Gov't]. 2009 Dec;36(12):1004-10.

[144] Bartold PM, Marino V, Cantley M, Haynes DR. Effect of Porphyromonas gingivalis-induced inflammation on the development of rheumatoid arthritis. *J Clin Periodontol.* [Research Support, Non-U.S. Gov't]. 2010 May;37(5):405-11.

[145] Cantley MD, Haynes DR, Marino V, Bartold PM. Pre-existing periodontitis exacerbates experimental arthritis in a mouse model. *J Clin Periodontol.* [Research Support, Non-U.S. Gov't]. 2011 Jun;38(6):532-41.

[146] Ogrendik M. Rheumatoid arthritis is an autoimmune disease caused by periodontal pathogens. *Int J Gen Med.* 2013;6:383-6.

[147] Zimmerli W, Trampuz A, Ochsner PE. Prosthetic-joint infections. *N Engl J Med.* [Review]. 2004 Oct 14;351(16):1645-54.

[148] Antibiotic prophylaxis for dental patients with total joint replacements. *J Am Dent Assoc.* [Guideline Patient Education Handout Practice Guideline]. 2003 Jul;134(7):895-9.

[149] Olsen I, Snorrason F, Lingaas E. Should patients with hip joint prosthesis receive antibiotic prophylaxis before dental treatment? *J Oral Microbiol.* 2010;2.

[150] Marek CL, Ernst EJ. The new American Academy of Orthopedic Surgeons' recommendations regarding antibiotic prophylaxis: where's the evidence? *Spec Care Dentist.* 2009 Nov-Dec;29(6):229-31.

[151] Uckay I, Pittet D, Bernard L, Lew D, Perrier A, Peter R. Antibiotic prophylaxis before invasive dental procedures in patients with arthroplasties of the hip and knee. *J Bone Joint Surg Br.* [Review]. 2008 Jul;90(7):833-8.

[152] Rubin R, Salvati EA, Lewis R. Infected total hip replacement after dental procedures. *Oral Surg Oral Med Oral Pathol.* [Case Reports]. 1976 Jan;41(1):18-23.

[153] Kaar TK, Bogoch ER, Devlin HR. Acute metastatic infection of a revision total hip arthroplasty with oral bacteria after noninvasive dental treatment. *J Arthroplasty.* [Case Reports]. 2000 Aug;15(5):675-8.

[154] Esposito S, Leone S. Prosthetic joint infections: microbiology, diagnosis, management and prevention. *Int J Antimicrob Agents.* [Review]. 2008 Oct;32(4):287-93.

[155] Assael LA. Oral bacteremia as a cause of prosthesis failure in patients with joint replacements. *J Oral Maxillofac Surg.* [Editorial]. 2009 Sep;67(9):1789-90.

[156] Ohyama H, Nakasho K, Yamanegi K, Noiri Y, Kuhara A, Kato-Kogoe N, et al. An unusual autopsy case of pyogenic liver abscess caused by periodontal bacteria. *Jpn J Infect Dis.* [Case Reports Research Support, Non-U.S. Gov't]. 2009 Sep;62(5):381-3.

[157] Rahamat-Langendoen JC, van Vonderen MG, Engstrom LJ, Manson WL, van Winkelhoff AJ, Mooi-Kokenberg EA. Brain abscess associated

with Aggregatibacter actinomycetemcomitans: case report and review of literature. *J Clin Periodontol.* [Case Reports Review]. 2011 Aug;38(8):702-6.

[158] Zijlstra EE, Swart GR, Godfroy FJ, Degener JE. Pericarditis, pneumonia and brain abscess due to a combined Actinomyces--Actinobacillus actinomycetemcomitans infection. *J Infect.* [Case Reports]. 1992 Jul;25(1):83-7.

[159] Kuijper EJ, Wiggerts HO, Jonker GJ, Schaal KP, de Gans J. Disseminated actinomycosis due to Actinomyces meyeri and Actinobacillus actinomycetemcomitans. *Scand J Infect Dis.* [Case Reports]. 1992;24(5):667-72.

[160] Kaplan AH, Weber DJ, Oddone EZ, Perfect JR. Infection due to Actinobacillus actinomycetemcomitans: 15 cases and review. *Rev Infect Dis.* [Case Reports Review]. 1989 Jan-Feb;11(1):46-63.

[161] Churton MC, Greer ND. Intracranial abscess secondary to dental infection. *N Z Dent J.* [Case Reports]. 1980 Apr;76(344):58-60.

[162] Garner JG. Isolation of Actinobacillus actinomycetemcomitans and Haemophilus aphrophilus at Auckland Hospital. *N Z Med J.* [Case Reports]. 1979 May 23;89(636):384-6.

[163] Ingham HR, Kalbag RM, Tharagonnet D, High AS, Sengupta RP, Selkon JB. Abscesses of the frontal lobe of the brain secondary to covert dental sepsis. *Lancet.* [Case Reports]. 1978 Sep 2;2(8088):497-9.

[164] Brewer NS, MacCarty CS, Wellman WE. Brain abscess: a review of recent experience. *Ann Intern Med.* 1975 Apr;82(4):571-6.

[165] Burgher LW, Loomis GW, Ware F. Systemic infection due to Actinobacillus actinomycetemcomitans. *Am J Clin Pathol.* 1973 Sep;60(3):412-5.

[166] Martin BF, Derby BM, Budzilovich GN, Ransohoff J. Brain abscess due to Actinobacillus actinomycetemcomitans. *Neurology.* 1967 Sep;17(9):833-7.

[167] Brook I, Frazier EH. The aerobic and anaerobic bacteriology of perirectal abscesses. *J Clin Microbiol.* 1997 Nov;35(11):2974-6.

[168] Lorenzo Garde L, Bolanos Rivero M, Turegano Garcia A, Martin Sanchez AM. [Intraperitoneal abscess for Eikenella corrodens]. *Rev Esp Quimioter.* [Case Reports Letter]. 2011 Jun;24(2):115-6.

[169] Danziger LH, Schoonover LL, Kale P, Resnick DJ. Eikenella corrodens as an intra-abdominal pathogen. *Am Surg.* [Case Reports Review]. 1994 Apr;60(4):296-9.

[170] Swidsinski A, Dorffel Y, Loening-Baucke V, Tertychnyy A, Biche-Ool S, Stonogin S, et al. Mucosal invasion by fusobacteria is a common feature of acute appendicitis in Germany, Russia, and China. *Saudi J Gastroenterol.* 2012 Jan-Feb;18(1):55-8.

[171] Swidsinski A, Dorffel Y, Loening-Baucke V, Theissig F, Ruckert JC, Ismail M, et al. Acute appendicitis is characterised by local invasion with Fusobacterium nucleatum/necrophorum. *Gut.* 2011 Jan;60(1):34-40.

[172] Tu YC, Lu MC, Chiang MK, Huang SP, Peng HL, Chang HY, et al. Genetic requirements for Klebsiella pneumoniae-induced liver abscess in an oral infection model. *Infect Immun.* [Research Support, Non-U.S. Gov't]. 2009 Jul;77(7):2657-71.

[173] Perez-Chaparro PJ, Lafaurie GI, Gracieux P, Meuric V, Tamanai-Shacoori Z, Castellanos JE, et al. Distribution of Porphyromonas gingivalis fimA genotypes in isolates from subgingival plaque and blood sample during bacteremia. *Biomedica.* [Comparative Study Research Support, Non-U.S. Gov't]. 2009 Jun;29(2):298-306.

[174] Perez-Chaparro PJ, Gracieux P, Lafaurie GI, Donnio PY, Bonnaure-Mallet M. Genotypic characterization of Porphyromonas gingivalis isolated from subgingival plaque and blood sample in positive bacteremia subjects with periodontitis. *J Clin Periodontol.* [Research Support, Non-U.S. Gov't]. 2008 Sep;35(9):748-53.

[175] Totaro MC, Cattani P, Ria F, Tolusso B, Gremese E, Fedele AL, et al. Porphyromonas gingivalis and the pathogenesis of rheumatoid arthritis: analysis of various compartments including the synovial tissue. *Arthritis Res Ther.* 2013 Jun 18;15(3):R66.

[176] Pucar A, Milasin J, Lekovic V, Vukadinovic M, Ristic M, Putnik S, et al. Correlation between atherosclerosis and periodontal putative pathogenic bacterial infections in coronary and internal mammary arteries. *J Periodontol.* [Research Support, Non-U.S. Gov't]. 2007 Apr;78(4):677-82.

[177] Ohki T, Itabashi Y, Kohno T, Yoshizawa A, Nishikubo S, Watanabe S, et al. Detection of periodontal bacteria in thrombi of patients with acute myocardial infarction by polymerase chain reaction. *Am Heart J.* [Comparative Study]. 2012 Feb;163(2):164-7.

[178] Chaparro A, Blanlot C, Ramirez V, Sanz A, Quintero A, Inostroza C, et al. Porphyromonas gingivalis, Treponema denticola and toll-like receptor 2 are associated with hypertensive disorders in placental tissue: a case-control study. *J Periodontal Res.* 2013 May 28.

[179] Swati P, Thomas B, Vahab SA, Kapaettu S, Kushtagi P. Simultaneous detection of periodontal pathogens in subgingival plaque and placenta of women with hypertension in pregnancy. *Arch Gynecol Obstet.* 2012 Mar;285(3):613-9.

[180] Ercan E, Eratalay K, Deren O, Gur D, Ozyuncu O, Altun B, et al. Evaluation of periodontal pathogens in amniotic fluid and the role of periodontal disease in pre-term birth and low birth weight. *Acta Odontol Scand.* [Research Support, Non-U.S. Gov't]. 2013 May-Jul;71(3-4): 553-9.

[181] Westling K, Vondracek M. Actinobacillus (Aggregatibacter) actinomycetemcomitans (HACEK) identified by PCR/16S rRNA sequence analysis from the heart valve in a patient with blood culture negative endocarditis. *Scand J Infect Dis.* [Case Reports]. 2008;40(11-12):981-3.

[182] Nakano K, Nemoto H, Nomura R, Inaba H, Yoshioka H, Taniguchi K, et al. Detection of oral bacteria in cardiovascular specimens. *Oral Microbiol Immunol.* [Research Support, Non-U.S. Gov't]. 2009 Feb;24(1):64-8.

[183] Okada M, Kobayashi T, Ito S, Yokoyama T, Komatsu Y, Abe A, et al. Antibody responses to periodontopathic bacteria in relation to rheumatoid arthritis in Japanese adults. *J Periodontol.* [Research Support, Non-U.S. Gov't]. 2011 Oct;82(10):1433-41.

[184] Stepanovic S, Tosic T, Savic B, Jovanovic M, K'Ouas G, Carlier JP. Brain abscess due to Actinobacillus actinomycetemcomitans. *Apmis.* [Case Reports]. 2005 Mar;113(3):225-8.

[185] Al Masalma M, Raoult D, Roux V. Phocaeicola abscessus gen. nov., sp. nov., an anaerobic bacterium isolated from a human brain abscess sample. *Int J Syst Evol Microbiol.* 2009 Sep;59(Pt 9):2232-7.

[186] Okuda K, Ishihara K, Nakagawa T, Hirayama A, Inayama Y. Detection of Treponema denticola in atherosclerotic lesions. *J Clin Microbiol.* [Research Support, Non-U.S. Gov't]. 2001 Mar;39(3):1114-7.

[187] Gonzalez Mera L, Fernandez Gonzalez S, Martinez Yelamos S, Fernandez Viladrich P. [Brain abscess caused by Eikenella corrodens and Streptococcus intermedius associated with bowel carcinoid tumour]. *Med Clin* (Barc). [Case Reports Letter]. 2005 Jun 18;125(3):117-8.

[188] Han YW, Shen T, Chung P, Buhimschi IA, Buhimschi CS. Uncultivated bacteria as etiologic agents of intra-amniotic inflammation leading to preterm birth. *J Clin Microbiol.* [Comparative Study Research Support, N.I.H., Extramural]. 2009 Jan;47(1):38-47.

[189] Wang X, Buhimschi CS, Temoin S, Bhandari V, Han YW, Buhimschi IA. Comparative microbial analysis of paired amniotic fluid and cord blood from pregnancies complicated by preterm birth and early-onset neonatal sepsis. *Plos One.* [Comparative Study Research Support, N.I.H., Extramural]. 2013;8(2):e56131.

[190] Han YW, Fardini Y, Chen C, Iacampo KG, Peraino VA, Shamonki JM, et al. Term stillbirth caused by oral Fusobacterium nucleatum. *Obstet Gynecol.* [Case Reports Research Support, N.I.H., Extramural]. 2010 Feb;115(2 Pt 2):442-5.

[191] Strauss J, Kaplan GG, Beck PL, Rioux K, Panaccione R, Devinney R, et al. Invasive potential of gut mucosa-derived Fusobacterium nucleatum positively correlates with IBD status of the host. *Inflamm Bowel Dis.* [Comparative Study Research Support, Non-U.S. Gov't]. 2011 Sep;17(9):1971-8.

[192] Temoin S, Chakaki A, Askari A, El-Halaby A, Fitzgerald S, Marcus RE, et al. Identification of oral bacterial DNA in synovial fluid of patients with arthritis with native and failed prosthetic joints. *J Clin Rheumatol.* [Research Support, N.I.H., Extramural Research Support, Non-U.S. Gov't]. 2012 Apr;18(3):117-21.

[193] Al Masalma M, Lonjon M, Richet H, Dufour H, Roche PH, Drancourt M, et al. Metagenomic analysis of brain abscesses identifies specific bacterial associations. *Clin Infect Dis.* [Research Support, Non-U.S. Gov't]. 2012 Jan 15;54(2):202-10.

[194] Heckmann JG, Lang CJ, Hartl H, Tomandl B. Multiple brain abscesses caused by Fusobacterium nucleatum treated conservatively. *Can J Neurol Sci.* [Case Reports]. 2003 Aug;30(3):266-8.

[195] Ismail Y, Mahendran V, Octavia S, Day AS, Riordan SM, Grimm MC, et al. Investigation of the enteric pathogenic potential of oral Campylobacter concisus strains isolated from patients with inflammatory bowel disease. *Plos One.* [Research Support, Non-U.S. Gov't]. 2012;7(5):e38217.

[196] Kinane DF, Riggio MP, Walker KF, MacKenzie D, Shearer B. Bacteraemia following periodontal procedures. *J Clin Periodontol.* [Research Support, Non-U.S. Gov't Research Support, U.S. Gov't, P.H.S.]. 2005 Jul;32(7):708-13.

[197] Gaetti-Jardim E, Jr., Marcelino SL, Feitosa AC, Romito GA, Avila-Campos MJ. Quantitative detection of periodontopathic bacteria in atherosclerotic plaques from coronary arteries. *J Med Microbiol.* [Research Support, Non-U.S. Gov't]. 2009 Dec;58(Pt 12):1568-75.

[198] Ng SC, Benjamin JL, McCarthy NE, Hedin CR, Koutsoumpas A, Plamondon S, et al. Relationship between human intestinal dendritic cells, gut microbiota, and disease activity in Crohn's disease. *Inflamm Bowel Dis*. [Comparative Study]. 2011 Oct;17(10):2027-37.

[199] Bahrani-Mougeot FK, Paster BJ, Coleman S, Ashar J, Knost S, Sautter RL, et al. Identification of oral bacteria in blood cultures by conventional versus molecular methods. *Oral Surg Oral Med Oral Pathol Oral Radiol Endod.* [Research Support, N.I.H., Extramural Research Support, Non-U.S. Gov't]. 2008 Jun;105(6):720-4.

[200] Tomas I, Alvarez M, Limeres J, Potel C, Medina J, Diz P. Prevalence, duration and aetiology of bacteraemia following dental extractions. *Oral Dis*. [Research Support, Non-U.S. Gov't]. 2007 Jan;13(1):56-62.

[201] Heimdahl A, Hall G, Hedberg M, Sandberg H, Soder PO, Tuner K, et al. Detection and quantitation by lysis-filtration of bacteremia after different oral surgical procedures. *J Clin Microbiol.* [Research Support, Non-U.S. Gov't]. 1990 Oct;28(10):2205-9.

[202] Morency AM, Rallu F, Laferriere C, Bujoldg E. Eradication of intra-amniotic Streptococcus mutans in a woman with a short cervix. *J Obstet Gynaecol Can.* [Case Reports Research Support, Non-U.S. Gov't]. 2006 Oct;28(10):898-902.

[203] van den Bogert B, Erkus O, Boekhorst J, de Goffau M, Smid EJ, Zoetendal EG, et al. Diversity of human small intestinal Streptococcus and Veillonella populations. *FEMS Microbiol Ecol.* [Research Support, Non-U.S. Gov't]. 2013 Aug;85(2):376-88.

[204] Kitten T, Munro CL, Zollar NQ, Lee SP, Patel RD. Oral streptococcal bacteremia in hospitalized patients: taxonomic identification and clinical characterization. *J Clin Microbiol.* [Research Support, N.I.H., Extramural]. 2012 Mar;50(3):1039-42.

[205] Huang IF, Chiou CC, Liu YC, Hsieh KS. Endocarditis caused by penicillin-resistant Streptococcus mitis in a 12-year-old boy. *J Microbiol Immunol Infect.* [Case Reports]. 2002 Jun;35(2):129-32.

[206] Saito N, Hida A, Koide Y, Ooka T, Ichikawa Y, Shimizu J, et al. Culture-negative brain abscess with Streptococcus intermedius infection with diagnosis established by direct nucleotide sequence analysis of the 16s ribosomal RNA gene. *Intern Med.* [Case Reports Research Support, Non-U.S. Gov't Review]. 2012;51(2):211-6.

[207] Inomata M, Ishihara Y, Matsuyama T, Imamura T, Maruyama I, Noguchi T, et al. Degradation of vascular endothelial thrombomodulin by arginine- and lysine-specific cysteine proteases from Porphyromonas

gingivalis. *J Periodontol.* [Research Support, Non-U.S. Gov't]. 2009 Sep;80(9):1511-7.

[208] Dietmann A, Millonig A, Combes V, Couraud PO, Kachlany SC, Grau GE. Effects of Aggregatibacter actinomycetemcomitans leukotoxin on endothelial cells. *Microb Pathog.* [Research Support, Non-U.S. Gov't]. 2013 Aug-Sep;61-62:43-50.

[209] Nakagawa I, Inaba H, Yamamura T, Kato T, Kawai S, Ooshima T, et al. Invasion of epithelial cells and proteolysis of cellular focal adhesion components by distinct types of Porphyromonas gingivalis fimbriae. *Infect Immun.* [Research Support, Non-U.S. Gov't]. 2006 Jul;74(7):3773-82.

[210] Kuboniwa M, Hasegawa Y, Mao S, Shizukuishi S, Amano A, Lamont RJ, et al. P. gingivalis accelerates gingival epithelial cell progression through the cell cycle. *Microbes Infect.* [Research Support, N.I.H., Extramural]. 2008 Feb;10(2):122-8.

[211] Nakhjiri SF, Park Y, Yilmaz O, Chung WO, Watanabe K, El-Sabaeny A, et al. Inhibition of epithelial cell apoptosis by Porphyromonas gingivalis. *FEMS Microbiol Lett.* [Research Support, U.S. Gov't, P.H.S.]. 2001 Jun 25;200(2):145-9.

[212] Paino A, Lohermaa E, Sormunen R, Tuominen H, Korhonen J, Pollanen MT, et al. Interleukin-1beta is internalised by viable Aggregatibacter actinomycetemcomitans biofilm and locates to the outer edges of nucleoids. *Cytokine.* 2012 Nov;60(2):565-74.

[213] Miles B, Zakhary I, El-Awady A, Scisci E, Carrion J, O'Neill JC, et al. SLO Homing Phenotype of Human Myeloid Dendritic cells Disrupted by an Intracellular Oral Pathogen. *Infect Immun.* 2013 Oct 14.

[214] Miyamoto T, Yumoto H, Takahashi Y, Davey M, Gibson FC, 3rd, Genco CA. Pathogen-accelerated atherosclerosis occurs early after exposure and can be prevented via immunization. *Infect Immun.* [Research Support, N.I.H., Extramural]. 2006 Feb;74(2):1376-80.

[215] Saadi-Thiers K, Huck O, Simonis P, Tilly P, Fabre JE, Tenenbaum H, et al. Periodontal and systemic responses in various mice models of experimental periodontitis: respective roles of inflammation duration and Porphyromonas gingivalis infection. *J Periodontol.* 2013 Mar;84(3):396-406.

[216] Kebschull M, Haupt M, Jepsen S, Deschner J, Nickenig G, Werner N. Mobilization of endothelial progenitors by recurrent bacteremias with a periodontal pathogen. *Plos One.* [Research Support, Non-U.S. Gov't]. 2013;8(1):e54860.

[217] Miyauchi S, Maekawa T, Aoki Y, Miyazawa H, Tabeta K, Nakajima T, et al. Oral infection with Porphyromonas gingivalis and systemic cytokine profile in C57BL/6.KOR-ApoE shl mice. J Periodontal Res. [Comparative Study Research Support, Non-U.S. Gov't]. 2012 Jun;47(3):402-8.

[218] Ashigaki N, Suzuki J, Ogawa M, Watanabe R, Aoyama N, Kobayashi N, et al. Periodontal bacteria aggravate experimental autoimmune myocarditis in mice. *Am J Physiol Heart Circ Physiol.* [Research Support, Non-U.S. Gov't]. 2013 Mar 1;304(5):H740-8.

[219] Kojima A, Nakano K, Wada K, Takahashi H, Katayama K, Yoneda M, et al. Infection of specific strains of Streptococcus mutans, oral bacteria, confers a risk of ulcerative colitis. *Sci Rep.* [Research Support, Non-U.S. Gov't]. 2012;2:332.

[220] Arce RM, Caron KM, Barros SP, Offenbacher S. Toll-like receptor 4 mediates intrauterine growth restriction after systemic Campylobacter rectus infection in mice. *Mol Oral Microbiol.* 2012 Oct;27(5):373-81.

[221] Nagata E, Okayama H, Ito HO, Yamashita Y, Inoue M, Oho T. Serotype-specific polysaccharide of Streptococcus mutans contributes to infectivity in endocarditis. *Oral Microbiol Immunol.* [Research Support, Non-U.S. Gov't]. 2006 Dec;21(6):420-3.

[222] Kunnen A, van Pampus M, Aarnoudse J, van der Schans C, Abbas F, Faas M. The effect of Porphyromonas gingivalis lipopolysaccharide on pregnancy in the rat. *Oral Dis.* 2013 Aug 20.

[223] Belanger M, Reyes L, von Deneen K, Reinhard MK, Progulske-Fox A, Brown MB. Colonization of maternal and fetal tissues by Porphyromonas gingivalis is strain-dependent in a rodent animal model. *Am J Obstet Gynecol.* [Research Support, Non-U.S. Gov't]. 2008 Jul;199(1):86 e1-7.

[224] Herzberg MC, Meyer MW. Effects of oral flora on platelets: possible consequences in cardiovascular disease. *J Periodontol.* [Research Support, Non-U.S. Gov't Research Support, U.S. Gov't, P.H.S.]. 1996 Oct;67(10 Suppl):1138-42.

[225] Zhang MZ, Li CL, Jiang YT, Jiang W, Sun Y, Shu R, et al. Porphyromonas gingivalis infection accelerates intimal thickening in iliac arteries in a balloon-injured rabbit model. *J Periodontol.* [Comparative Study Research Support, Non-U.S. Gov't]. 2008 Jul;79(7):1192-9.

[226] Boggess KA, Madianos PN, Preisser JS, Moise KJ, Jr., Offenbacher S. Chronic maternal and fetal Porphyromonas gingivalis exposure during

pregnancy in rabbits. *Am J Obstet Gynecol.* [Research Support, U.S. Gov't, P.H.S.]. 2005 Feb;192(2):554-7.

[227] Imamura T, Pike RN, Potempa J, Travis J. Pathogenesis of periodontitis: a major arginine-specific cysteine proteinase from Porphyromonas gingivalis induces vascular permeability enhancement through activation of the kallikrein/kinin pathway. *J Clin Invest.* [Research Support, U.S. Gov't, P.H.S.]. 1994 Jul;94(1):361-7.

[228] Newnham JP, Shub A, Jobe AH, Bird PS, Ikegami M, Nitsos I, et al. The effects of intra-amniotic injection of periodontopathic lipopolysaccharides in sheep. *Am J Obstet Gynecol.* [Comparative Study Research Support, N.I.H., Extramural Research Support, Non-U.S. Gov't Research Support, U.S. Gov't, P.H.S.]. 2005 Aug;193(2):313-21.

[229] Ebersole JL, Cappelli D, Mathys EC, Steffen MJ, Singer RE, Montgomery M, et al. Periodontitis in humans and non-human primates: oral-systemic linkage inducing acute phase proteins. *Ann Periodontol.* [Research Support, N.I.H., Extramural Research Support, Non-U.S. Gov't Research Support, U.S. Gov't, P.H.S.]. 2002 Dec;7(1):102-11.

[230] Ebersole JL, Cappelli D, Mott G, Kesavalu L, Holt SC, Singer RE. Systemic manifestations of periodontitis in the non-human primate. *J Periodontal Res.* [Research Support, Non-U.S. Gov't]. 1999 Oct;34(7):358-62.

[231] Ebersole JL, Steffen MJ, Holt SC, Kesavalu L, Chu L, Cappelli D. Systemic inflammatory responses in progressing periodontitis during pregnancy in a baboon model. *Clin Exp Immunol.* [Research Support, N.I.H., Extramural Research Support, U.S. Gov't, P.H.S.]. 2010 Dec;162(3):550-9.

In: Bacteremia
Editor: Jodie P. Williams

ISBN: 978-1-63117-290-8

Chapter II

Lactobacillemia: Epidemiolgy, Clinical Features, Diagnosis and Treatment

Suresh Antony[1]* and Delfina C. Dominguez[2]
[1]Department of Clinical Laboratory Science, El Paso, TX, US
[2]Paul F. Foster School of Medicine, Texas Tech University Health Science Center, The University of Texas at El Paso, TX, US

Abstract

Lactobacillemia is a rare cause of bacteremia and the true clinical significance of this entity is just being delineated. *Lactobacillus* is a gram-positive bacillus that is for the most part intrinsically resistant to vancomycin but appears to be susceptible to most beta-lactams, erythromycin and clindamycin. *Lactobacilli* are a part of the normal gastrointestinal and genitourinary flora and for many years was regarded as non-pathogenic. There have been several case reports of *Lactobacillus* causing infections such as bacteremia, abscesses, peritonitis, meningitis and endocarditis.

L. rhamonosus, L. acidophilus and *L. casei* seem to have been implicated in a variety of infections. Interestingly, pre-administration of

* Corresponding author: Suresh J. Antony MD, 1205 N. Oregon, El Paso, Texas 79902, Email: suresh.antony@att.net, Tel; 915-5335900, Fax 915-5334902.

commercially available probiotics seem to have been implicated in sepsis in some of these cases. Lactobacillemia may be seen as an isolated infection or more often, as a poly-microbial infection. It tends to occur in patients who have been treated with antibiotics that have no activity on *Lactobacillus.* Many of the patients described in the literature are immuno-compromised with underling disease processes such as cancer, recent surgery, diabetes, and immunosuppressive therapy. However, patients with normal immune systems and *Lactobacillus* infection have also been described in the literature. Diagnosis is usually made on the isolation of the pathogens on blood cultures but more recently can be made using a rapid molecular method using terminal restriction fragment polymorphism analysis of the 16S rRNA gene. Some interesting questions still remain to be addressed such as recommendations in the use of prophylactic *Lactobacillus* on diseases such as irritable bowel syndrome, *Clostridium difficile* colitis and even routine use of this supplement and the risk of bacteremia.

Introduction

Lactobacillus species are ubiquitous microorganisms colonizing the mucosal surface of the mouth, gastrointestinal tract and genitourinary tract. This bacterium has increasingly been reported as a cause of serious infections in both immunocompetent and immunocompromised hosts. [1-9]. Serious infections caused *Lactobacillus* infections include bacterial endocarditis however lactobacillus has been reported as a cause of septicemia as well [1, 5, 10-12]. Even though infections associated with probiotic strains of *Lactobacilli* are extremely rare, cases of Lactobacilli sepsis linked to probiotic therapy have been reported [13-15].

This article reviews the clinical features, laboratory characteristics and treatment of patients with Lactobacillemia.

Microbiology

The genus *Lactobacillus* is a Gram positive, catalase negative bacteria that belongs to the family *Lactobacillaceae*. Taxonomically these organisms are very diverse. At present, the genus comprises of 152 species, and based on 16S rRNA analysis the family has been divided into 15 groups [16]. These bacteria are generally characterized by having a low GC content. *Lactobacilli* are nutritionally fastidious and have a fermentative metabolism producing lactic acid as the major end product [17]. Species of the genus *Lactobacillus* have been extensively studied in food microbiology, industrial applications and human nutrition. These organisms have been used in food preservation, starters for dairy products, fermented vegetables, wine and beer industry, silage inoculants and for potential production of 1,3-propanediol, a key component of polymer business [18, 19]. Members of the genus *Lactobacillus* are ubiquitous found in humans and a variety of plants and animals. *Lactobacillus* species are commensals of human mucosal tissue including the oropharynx, vagina and the gut. *Lactobacillus* vary in morphology sometimes appearing as rods or coccobacilli. Thus, these organisms can be confused with other genera including *Corynebacterium, Clostridium Nocardia* and *Streptococcus.* The lack of motility and catalase negativity distinguish *Lactobacillus* from *Listeria monocytogenes* and a negative hydrogen sulfide reaction distinguishes them from *Erysipelothrix rusopathie.* [5]. Routine identification of *Lactobacilli* to the species level is rarely done due to media availability and because the identification is a time consuming process. *Lactobacillus* species most frequently isolated from disease include *L. casei, L. acidophilus and L. rhamnosus.* Most frequent concomitant organisms in Lactobacillus polymicrbial infections include: *Enterococci, Pseudomonas aeruginosa, Klebsiella oxytoca, Streptococcus viridans, coagulase-negative Staphylococcus, Candida krusei and Torulopsis glabrata* [1, 2, 5].

Epidemiology

The association of lactobacillemia with other polymicrobial infections has been documented in some series [2, 5, 20, 21]. The reason for this presentation is not clear. Most infections occur in immunosuppressed patients or patients with underlying disease such as diabetes, malignancy, transplant patients, previous broad spectrum antibiotic therapy and in patients with surgical interventions [4, 5, 10, 12, 22, 23]. However, *Lactobacillus* bacteremia has also been reported in immunocompetent individuals [8]. The age range of patients with lactobacillemia is broad including children, adolescents and adults [4, 10, 24]. Approximately, 51% of the patients had received antibiotics prior to developing lactobacillemia [5]. The use of vancomycin has been associated to *Lactobacillus* bacteremia. It is proposed that vancomycin could favor the emergence and persistence of the organism since several *Lactobacilli species* are intrinsically resistant to the antibiotic. [25, 26]. Lactobacillemia clinical features range from asymptomatic to severe septicemia, and may be presented with a wide variety of clinical syndromes including: bacteremia, endocarditis, urinary tract infections, meningitis, dental infections, intra-abdominal and liver abscesses [24, 26-30]. According to Cannon et al., the mortality rate of lactobacillemia has been reported to be of about 30%.

Risk Factors

The risk factors for the development of Lactobacillemia appear to be immunocompromised conditions and include persistent prolonged neutropenia, the use of broad-spectrum antibiotics especially vancomycin which, results in persistence of resistant gastrointestinal flora and other immunosuppressive conditions. [1, 5, 7, 11, 12, 21]. Approximately 40% of the patients had underlying malignancy, 75% had previous antimicrobial therapy, 38% had undergone surgeries, 22-27% had diabetes mellitus or had received corticosteroids, and 5% of the patients had undergone organ transplantation [1, 4, 5, 10, 12, 21]. Selected bowel decontamination which, is used in some liver transplant recipients and the use of Roux-en-may play a role by altering the bowel flora resulting in *Lactobacillus* bacteremia [12]. In cancer patients, it appears to be more common in patients with acute myelogenous leukemia (5.4%). Additionally, other risk factors in neutropenic patients include mucositis, and previous antibiotic therapy [3, 11].

Clinical Features

The clinical presentation of Lactobacillemia may be highly variable due to a number of factors including: virulence of the pathogen, portal of entry, host susceptibility, and evolution of the condition [31-33].

Patients with lactobacillus bacteremia in the absence of endocarditis may present with a wide range of clinical features ranging from asymptomatic to a sepsis- like syndrome. The patient average age is between 55-60 years with no gender predisposition. The average duration of hospitalization is between 10 - 14 days, with an average duration of antibiotic treatment of 12 days. [1, 2, 5, 21]. Multiple portals of entries have been described including the oropharynx, genitourinary tract and gastrointestinal tract.

Lactobacillus endocarditis has been reported in >41 patients [7, 34]. This entity has occurred in both native and prosthetic valves. The clinical presentation of *Lactobacillus* endocarditis is similar to that of other pathogenic bacteria without any classical features. It appears that the clinical cure can be achieved in most cases with valve replacement needed in only a small proportion of the cases. Treatment failures occur when patients are not treated with a combination of penicillin and aminoglycoside but with the beta-lactams alone. [7, 21]. Vancomycin and cephalosporin's are not good options due to the intrinsic antimicrobial resistance to these drugs. In endocarditis associated bacteremia 80% of the cases are subacute with a time frame of 4 weeks before actual diagnosis, recent oropharyngeal manipulations with 60 % having previous cardiac abnormalities. Mitral/aortic valves seem to be the most affected. The majority of the cases appeared to be native valves with only a few being prosthetic. There also appeared to be a higher rate of systemic embolization to the brain and aortofemoral vessals (55%). In addition, there appears to be a higher failure rate in the treatment of patients with endocarditis with penicillin despite the use of high doses of penicillin (24 million units/day). Cure was achieved when the dose was raised to 48 million units/day or when combined with another antibiotic for synergistic effect (streptomycin or gentamicin) [21]. It appears that the *in vitro* synergism demonstrated to be useful and should be used to guide treatment, and that the Minimum Bactericidal Concentration (MBC) may be used to guide treatment.

Lactobacillemia in AIDS

There have been 4 patients reported in the literature. They shared some common characteristics. Advanced AIDS with CD4 count <55 cells/μl, all had Groshong catheters which, were not infected, all had concomitant coagulase-negative *Staphyloccous* bacteremia, and the majority had received vancomycin prior to the onset of Lactobacillemia [23, 35]. Signs and symptoms of *Lactobacillus* bacteremia included fever (60-100%) leukocytosis (22%) and rigors (22%). Unusual presentations included hypothermia and leukopenia.

Diagnosis of Lactobacillemia

The criteria used to diagnose Lactobacillemia includes recovering the organism from at least two sets of blood cultures or the isolation of the *Lactobacillus* species from blood, tissue or other material obtained from the site of infection [1]. These standards assure that the organism recovered is indeed the etiologic agent rather than a contaminant. There is no evidence that *Lactobacillus* species are part of the skin flora. In a comprehensive analysis of 500 episodes of bacteremia, Weinstein and coworkers did not find Lactobacillus species as contaminants. These findings support the fact that Lactobacillus bacteremia is a true infection when detected.

Identification of *Lactobacillus* isolates to the species level is rarely done in routine laboratory practice, mainly because *Lactobacillus* is normal flora generally considered a contaminant, and because its identification is cumbersome. In addition, most of the conventional methods for identification, Vitek, Microscan and API systems may give inconclusive results or identify the organism only at the Genus level [4, 8, 30]. However, phenotypic identification of some Lactobacillus species have been successfully identified using API 50CH test kit and API CHL medium (bioMérieux) [36]. Another factor that may complicate the identification process is the variable microscopic morphology of *Lactobacilli*, which may be confused with *Streptococci*, *Corynebacterium* and/or *Clostridia* [37, 38].

Therefore, confirmation of *Lactobacillus* bacteremia is done by molecular methods. PCR and sequencing of the 16S rRNA gene is the method most commonly used for Lactobacillus species identification [5, 8, 14, 29, 36, 38]. Pulse field Gel Electrophoresis (PFGE) and DNA fingerprinting have been used to perform strain comparisons [14, 29]. Despite the high capabilities of DNA amplification technology, Gouriet et al., experienced difficulties discriminating among *Lactobacilli* species and they used matrix-assisted laser desorption/ionization time-of-flight mass spectrometry (MALDI-TOF MS) [4]. This method identifies bacteria by analysis of protein profiles derived from highly conserved proteins. The protein profile can be obtained by a bacterial protein extract or by direct ionization of a colony. Identificatoin is done after the protein profile obtained is compared to a database of protein profiles from reference strains. Currently MALDI-TOF MS requires culturing of the organism prior to identification [39]. However, there are reports that showed promising results without the need to subculture [40-42].

Antimicrobial susceptibility of *Lactobacillus* is species dependent. While *L. delbrüeckii* and *L. acidophilus* group are susceptible to most antibiotics, *L. casei*, *L. rhamnosus*, *L. fermentum* and *L. curvatus* are intrinsically resistant to glycopeptides [43]. Most clinical isolates reported showed low MICs to imipenem, pipericillin, tazobactam, erythromycin and clindamycin. Susceptibility to penicillin and cephalosporins has been reported to vary among species [29]. E-test, microdilution and disc diffusion methods have been used to perform antimicrobial susceptibility in *Lactobacilli*.

Probiotics and Its Possible Relationship to Lactobacullus Infections

Probiotics have been defined as non-pathogenic microorganisms that when ingested exert a positive influence on host health or physiology. [44]. They consist of lactic acid bacteria, bifidobacteria, and yeasts (*Saccharomyces*), and may be present in either food, food supplements or in drugs. The mechanism of action is believed to be either through direct modifications of the endogenous flora or it could be an indirect interaction through immunomodulation [45-47]. The active components are thought to be bacterial formylated peptides, peptidoglycan cell wall constituents and nucleotides [48]. Even though Lactobacillus infections due to probiotic organisms are rare there is controversy and debate about the clinical significance of *Lactobacillus* bacteremia caused by probiotic organisms. One of the first cases of probiotic related infections was reported in a patient with a liver abscess with *L. rhamonosus* GG, a well-studied probiotic strain [49]. Since then there have been several cases associated to *Lactobacillus* infections including endocarditis, pneumonia, deep abscesses, bacteremia and other conditions [4, 13, 14, 25, 37, 50, 51]. Studies have been done where *Lactobacillus* species causing bacteremia have been characterized to the species level. These studies have reported that a number of Lactobacilli strains isolated from blood samples were indistinguishable from the probiotic strain *L. rhamnosus* GG. Predisposing factors to the bacteremia were immunosuppression, underlying disease prolong hospitalization [14, 15, 26, 28, 51]. Identification of Lactobacilli has been than by molecular technology since More conventional methods, API 50CH, BACTEC, MicroScan and Vitek are not able to discriminate accurately among species [4, 8, 14, 28, 36].

As probiotic Lactobacilli are increasing used it is important to keep in mind that also there is increased used of immunosuppressive therapy, prolong antibiotics, which may be ineffective against Lactobacilli and may enhance the possibility of these organisms to cause invasive disease.

Treatment

Susceptibility Testing

The treatment of Lactobacillemia should be guided by the clinical presentation and the results of susceptibility testing because of the unusual antimicrobial susceptibility associated with this pathogen [12, 21]. Several investigators have reported vancomycin resistance with MIC's of more than 256 μg per ML. The frequent use of vancomycin therapy for patients in intensive care units and in neutropenic patients may account for the pathogenic characteristic of this organism in this patient population [21, 52, 53]. The mechanism of vancomycin resistance is not known it may involve diminished binding of the antibiotic to the cell wall as a result of altered peptide sequences or the activity of vancomycin may be reduced by exclusion of its target sites for the target cell wall [54].

Much of the early literature supported the use of a combination of penicillin or other beta-lactam agents and an aminoglycoside in the treatment of Lactobacillemia especially when deep-seated infection was suspected [21, 55]. Bayer and colleagues noted that the MIC's of penicillin, ampicillin and cephalothin for 9 isolates were within achievable serum levels of these drugs. However, only 52% of MBC's of these three antimicrobials where within the range of achievable serum levels. He also noted synergistic activity of penicillin and ampicillin with either streptomycin or gentamicin but no synergy was noted between vancomycin and the aminoglycosides [21]. Of the parental cephalosporin's, cephaloridine, cefazolin and cefamandole have the most inhibitory and bactericidal capability. These studies also demonstrated that the Lactobacillus would generally resistant to metronidazole, norfloxacin and ciprofloxacin as well as trimethoprim sulfamethoxazole. The third-generation cephalosporins appear to vary in the effectiveness against these isolates. Clindamycin gentamicin, tobramycin, chloramphenicol were almost 100% effective [12, 21, 54, 56]. These studies also show the MIC's of ampicillin were in the range of 1-2 μg per ML. Thus large intravenous doses of penicillin would be necessary to effectively inhibit lactobacillus. The MIC's of imipenem and erythromycin were low, however these agents have been used to treat three patients with lactobacillus bacteremia and proved to be a useful therapeutic alternative for patients with penicillin allergy. Although further studies are indicated to confirm these data given the unusual invariable sensitivities reported in the literature, it is obvious that sensitivity testing is of utmost clinical importance in lactobacillus septicemia.

Conclusion

In summary, Lactobacillus is becoming an increasingly important pathogen associated with both immunocompromised and immunocompetent patients. Identification and susceptibility testing of gram-positive rods isolated from the bloodstream of septic patients will aid in the diagnosis and management of this condition. Lactobacillus appears to be uniformly resistant to vancomycin and variably resistant to the cephalosporins and quinolones. Antimicrobials of choice include erythromycin, penicillin, clindamycin aminoglycosides and imipenem. Combination therapy should be the standard of care in endocarditis and possibly other deep-seated infections.

References

[1] Antony, SJ. Lactobacillemia: an emerging cause of infection in both the immunocompromised and the immunocompetent host. *Journal of the National Medical Association*. 2000 Feb, 92(2), 83-6. PubMed PMID: 10800296. Pubmed Central PMCID: 2640534.

[2] Antony, SJ; Stratton, CW; Dummer, JS. Lactobacillus bacteremia: description of the clinical course in adult patients without endocarditis. *Clin Infect Dis.*, 1996 Oct, 23(4), 773-8. PubMed PMID: 8909843.

[3] Cooper, BA. Superiority of simplified assay for folate with Lactobacillus casei ATCC 7469 over assay with chloramphenicol-adapted strain. *Journal of clinical pathology.*, 1973 Dec, 26(12), 963-7. PubMed PMID: 4206241. Pubmed Central PMCID: 477938.

[4] Gouriet, F; Million, M; Henri, M; Fournier, PE; Raoult, D. Lactobacillus rhamnosus bacteremia: an emerging clinical entity. *Eur J Clin Microbiol Infect Dis.*, 2012 Sep, 31(9), 2469-80. PubMed PMID: 22544343.

[5] Husni, RN; Gordon, SM; Washington, JA; Longworth, DL. Lactobacillus bacteremia and endocarditis: review of 45 cases. *Clin Infect Dis*. 1997 Nov, 25(5), 1048-55. PubMed PMID: 9402355.

[6] Schoon, Y; Schuurman, B; Buiting, AG; Kranendonk, SE; Graafsma, SJ. Aortic graft infection by Lactobacillus casei: a case report. *The Netherlands journal of medicine*., 1998 Feb, 52(2), 71-4. PubMed PMID: 9557529.

[7] Sussman, JI; Baron, EJ; Goldberg, SM; Kaplan, MH; Pizzarello, RA. Clinical manifestations and therapy of Lactobacillus endocarditis: report of a case and review of the literature. *Reviews of infectious diseases*., 1986 Sep-Oct, 8(5), 771-6. PubMed PMID: 3097786.

[8] Tommasi, C; Equitani, F; Masala, M; Ballardini, M; Favaro, M; Meledandri, M; et al. Diagnostic difficulties of Lactobacillus casei bacteraemia in immunocompetent patients: a case report. *Journal of medical case reports*., 2008, 2, 315. PubMed PMID: 18826603. Pubmed Central PMCID: 2566577.

[9] Saxelin, M; Chuang, NH; Chassy, B; Rautelin, H; Makela, PH; Salminen, S; et al. Lactobacilli and bacteremia in southern Finland, 1989-1992. *Clin Infect Dis*., 1996 Mar, 22(3), 564-6. PubMed PMID: 8852980. Epub 1996/03/01. eng.

[10] Cannon, JP; Lee, TA; Bolanos, JT; Danziger, LH. Pathogenic relevance of Lactobacillus: a retrospective review of over 200 cases. *Eur J Clin Microbiol Infect Dis*., 2005 Jan, 24(1), 31-40. PubMed PMID: 15599646.

[11] Fruchart, C; Salah, A; Gray, C; Martin, E; Stamatoullas, A; Bonmarchand, G; et al. Lactobacillus species as emerging pathogens in neutropenic patients. *Eur J Clin Microbiol Infect Dis*., 1997 Sep, 16(9), 681-4. PubMed PMID: 9352263.

[12] Patel, HM; Wang, R; Chandrashekar, O; Pandiella, SS; Webb, C. Proliferation of Lactobacillus plantarum in solid-state fermentation of oats. *Biotechnology progress*., 2004 Jan-Feb, 20(1), 110-6. PubMed PMID: 14763831.

[13] Kunz, AN; Noel, JM; Fairchok, MP. Two cases of Lactobacillus bacteremia during probiotic treatment of short gut syndrome. *Journal of pediatric gastroenterology and nutrition*., 2004 Apr, 38(4), 457-8. PubMed PMID: 15085028.

[14] Land, MH; Rouster-Stevens, K; Woods, CR; Cannon, ML; Cnota, J; Shetty, AK. Lactobacillus sepsis associated with probiotic therapy. *Pediatrics*., 2005 Jan, 115(1), 178-81. PubMed PMID: 15629999.

[15] Vahabnezhad, E; Mochon, AB; Wozniak, LJ; Ziring, DA. Lactobacillus bacteremia associated with probiotic use in a pediatric patient with ulcerative colitis. *Journal of clinical gastroenterology.*, 2013 May-Jun, 47(5), 437-9. PubMed PMID: 23426446.

[16] Salvetti, E; Torriani, S; Felis, GE. The Genus Lactobacillus: A Taxonomic Update. *Probiotics and Antimicrobial Proteins.*, 2012, 4, 217-26.

[17] Canchaya, C; Claesson, MJ; Fitzgerald, GF; van, Sinderen, D; O'Toole, PW. Diversity of the genus Lactobacillus revealed by comparative genomics of five species. *Microbiology.*, 2006 Nov, 152(Pt 11), 3185-96. PubMed PMID: 17074890.

[18] Giraffa, G; Chanishvili, N; Widyastuti, Y. Importance of lactobacilli in food and feed biotechnology. *Research in microbiology.*, 2010 Jul-Aug, 161(6), 480-7. PubMed PMID: 20302928.

[19] Nakamura, CE; Whited, GM. Metabolic engineering for the microbial production of 1,3-propanediol. *Current opinion in biotechnology.*, 2003 Oct, 14(5), 454-9. PubMed PMID: 14580573.

[20] Arpi, M; Vancanneyt, M; Swings, J; Leisner, JJ. Six cases of Lactobacillus bacteraemia: identification of organisms and antibiotic susceptibility and therapy. *Scandinavian journal of infectious diseases.*, 2003, 35(6-7), 404-8. PubMed PMID: 12953954.

[21] Bayer, AS; Chow, AW; Concepcion, NF; Guze, LB. Comparative *in vitro* activity of five cephalosporins against Lactobacilli. *Antimicrobial agents and chemotherapy.*, 1979 Jul, 16(1), 112-3. PubMed PMID: 475370. Pubmed Central PMCID: 352801.

[22] Toporoff, B; Rosado, LJ; Appleton, CP; Sethi, GK; Copeland, JG. Successful treatment of early infective endocarditis and mediastinitis in a heart transplant recipient. *The Journal of heart and lung transplantation: the official publication of the International Society for Heart Transplantation.*, 1994 May-Jun, 13(3), 546-8. PubMed PMID: 8061034.

[23] Horwitch, CA; Furseth, HA; Larson, AM; Jones, TL; Olliffe, JF; Spach, DH. Lactobacillemia in three patients with AIDS. *Clin Infect Dis.*, 1995 Dec, 21(6), 1460-2. PubMed PMID: 8749632. Epub 1995/12/01. eng.

[24] Lee, AC; Siao-Ping, Ong, ND. Food-borne bacteremic illnesses in febrile neutropenic children. *Hematol Rep.*, 2011 Aug 31, 3(2), e11. PubMed PMID: 22184532. Pubmed Central PMCID: 3238479. Epub 2011/12/21. eng.

[25] Olano, A; Chua, J; Schroeder, S; Minari, A; La, Salvia, M; Hall, G. Weissella confusa (basonym: Lactobacillus confusus) bacteremia: a case report. *J Clin Microbiol.*, 2001 Apr, 39(4), 1604-7. PubMed PMID: 11283096. Pubmed Central PMCID: 87979.

[26] Robin, F; Paillard, C; Marchandin, H; Demeocq, F; Bonnet, R; Hennequin, C. Lactobacillus rhamnosus meningitis following recurrent episodes of bacteremia in a child undergoing allogeneic hematopoietic stem cell transplantation. *J Clin Microbiol.*, 2010 Nov, 48(11), 4317-9. PubMed PMID: 20844225. Pubmed Central PMCID: 3020890.

[27] Chazan, B; Raz, R; Shental, Y; Sprecher, H; Colodner, R. Bacteremia and pyelonephritis caused by Lactobacillus jensenii in a patient with urolithiasis. *The Israel Medical Association journal: IMAJ.*, 2008 Feb, 10(2), 164-5. PubMed PMID: 18432039.

[28] Salminen, MK; Rautelin, H; Tynkkynen, S; Poussa, T; Saxelin, M; Valtonen, V; et al. Lactobacillus bacteremia, clinical significance, and patient outcome, with special focus on probiotic L. rhamnosus GG. *Clin Infect Dis.*, 2004 Jan 1, 38(1), 62-9. PubMed PMID: 14679449.

[29] Salminen, MK; Rautelin, H; Tynkkynen, S; Poussa, T; Saxelin, M; Valtonen, V; et al. Lactobacillus bacteremia, species identification, and antimicrobial susceptibility of 85 blood isolates. *Clin Infect Dis.*, 2006 Mar 1, 42(5), e35-44. PubMed PMID: 16447101.

[30] Suarez-Garcia, I; Sanchez-Garcia, A; Soler, L; Malmierca, E; Gomez-Cerezo, J. Lactobacillus jensenii bacteremia and endocarditis after dilatation and curettage: case report and literature review. *Infection.*, 2012 Apr, 40(2), 219-22. PubMed PMID: 21866337.

[31] Lever, A; Mackenzie, I. Sepsis: definition, epidemiology, and diagnosis. *Bmj.*, 2007 Oct 27, 335(7625), 879-83. PubMed PMID: 17962288. Pubmed Central PMCID: 2043413.

[32] Angus, DC; Wax, RS. Epidemiology of sepsis: an update. *Crit Care Med.*, 2001 Jul, 29(7 Suppl), S109-16. PubMed PMID: 11445744. Epub 2001/07/11. eng.

[33] Flaws, ML. *Bacteremia and Sepsis.* In: Mahon CR, Lehman DC, Manuselis G, editors. *Diagnostic Microbiology.*, 4th ed. Maryland Heights. MO: WB Saunders Company; 2011.

[34] Griffiths, JK; Daly, JS; Dodge, RA. Two cases of endocarditis due to Lactobacillus species: antimicrobial susceptibility, review, and discussion of therapy. *Clin Infect Dis.*, 1992 Aug, 15(2), 250-5. PubMed PMID: 1520759.

[35] Sherman, JM; Hodge, HM. The Value of Certain Tests in the Differentiation of Lactobacillus bulgaricus from Lactobacillus acidophilus. *Journal of bacteriology.*, 1940 Jul, 40(1), 11-22. PubMed PMID: 16560332. Pubmed Central PMCID: 374618.

[36] Wallet, F; Dessein, R; Armand, S; Courcol, RJ. Molecular diagnosis of endocarditis due to Lactobacillus casei subsp. rhamnosus. *Clin Infect Dis.*, 2002 Nov 15, 35(10), e117-9. PubMed PMID: 12410496.

[37] Harlan, NP; Kempker, RR; Parekh, SM; Burd, EM; Kuhar, DT. Weissella confusa bacteremia in a liver transplant patient with hepatic artery thrombosis. *Transplant infectious disease: an official journal of the Transplantation Society.*, 2011 Jun, 13(3), 290-3. PubMed PMID: 21504525.

[38] Russo, A; Angeletti, S; Lorino, G; Venditti, C; Falcone, M; Dicuonzo, G; et al. A case of Lactobacillus casei bacteraemia associated with aortic dissection: is there a link? *The new microbiologica.*, 2010 Apr, 33(2), 175-8. PubMed PMID: 20518281.

[39] Wolk, DM; Dunne, WM. New Technologies in Clinical Microbiology. *Journal of Clinical Microbiology.*, 2011, 49(9), S62-S7.

[40] Moussaoui, W; Jaulhac, B; Hoffmann, AM; Ludes, B; Kostrzewa, M; Riegel, P; et al. Matrix-assisted laser desorption ionization time-of-flight mass spectrometry identifies 90% of bacteria directly from blood culture vials. *Clinical microbiology and infection: the official publication of the European Society of Clinical Microbiology and Infectious Diseases.*, 2010 Nov, 16(11), 1631-8. PubMed PMID: 20825442.

[41] Stevenson, LG; Drake, SK; Murray, PR. Rapid identification of bacteria in positive blood culture broths by matrix-assisted laser desorption ionization-time of flight mass spectrometry. *J Clin Microbiol.*, 2010 Feb, 48(2), 444-7. PubMed PMID: 19955282. Pubmed Central PMCID: 2815598.

[42] Prod'hom, G; Bizzini, A; Durussel, C; Bille, J; Greub, G. Matrix-assisted laser desorption ionization-time of flight mass spectrometry for direct bacterial identification from positive blood culture pellets. *J Clin Microbiol.*, 2010 Apr, 48(4), 1481-3. PubMed PMID: 20164269. Pubmed Central PMCID: 2849571. Epub 2010/02/19. eng.

[43] Danielsen, M; Wind, A. Susceptibility of Lactobacillus spp. to antimicrobial agents. *International journal of food microbiology.*, 2003 Jan 26, 82(1), 1-11. PubMed PMID: 12505455.

[44] Schrezenmeir, J; de, Vrese, M. Probiotics, prebiotics, and synbiotics--approaching a definition. *The American journal of clinical nutrition.*, 2001 Feb, 73(2 Suppl), 361S-4S. PubMed PMID: 11157342.

[45] Isolauri, E; Arvola, T; Sutas, Y; Moilanen, E; Salminen, S. Probiotics in the management of atopic eczema. *Clin Exp Allergy.*, 2000 Nov, 30(11), 1604-10. PubMed PMID: 11069570. Epub 2000/11/09. eng.

[46] Kalliomaki, M; Salminen, S; Arvilommi, H; Kero, P; Koskinen, P; Isolauri, E. Probiotics in primary prevention of atopic disease: a randomised placebo-controlled trial. *Lancet.*, 2001 Apr 7, 357(9262), 1076-9. PubMed PMID: 11297958. Epub 2001/04/12. eng.

[47] Majamaa, H; Isolauri, E. Probiotics: a novel approach in the management of food allergy. *J Allergy Clin Immunol.*, 1997 Feb, 99(2), 179-85. PubMed PMID: 9042042. Epub 1997/02/01. eng.

[48] Marteau, P; Shanahan, F. Basic aspects and pharmacology of probiotics: an overview of pharmacokinetics, mechanisms of action and side-effects. *Best practice & research Clinical gastroenterology.*, 2003 Oct, 17(5), 725-40. PubMed PMID: 14507584.

[49] Rautio, M; Jousimies-Somer, H; Kauma, H; Pietarinen, I; Saxelin, M; Tynkkynen, S; et al. Liver abscess due to a Lactobacillus rhamnosus strain indistinguishable from L. rhamnosus strain GG. *Clin Infect Dis.*, 1999 May, 28(5), 1159-60. PubMed PMID: 10452653.

[50] Mackay, AD; Taylor, MB; Kibbler, CC; Hamilton-Miller, JM. Lactobacillus endocarditis caused by a probiotic organism. *Clinical microbiology and infection: the official publication of the European Society of Clinical Microbiology and Infectious Diseases.*, 1999 May, 5(5), 290-2. PubMed PMID: 11856270.

[51] Salminen, MK; Tynkkynen, S; Rautelin, H; Saxelin, M; Vaara, M; Ruutu, P; et al. Lactobacillus bacteremia during a rapid increase in probiotic use of Lactobacillus rhamnosus GG in Finland. *Clin Infect Dis.*, 2002 Nov 15, 35(10), 1155-60. PubMed PMID: 12410474.

[52] Andriessen, MP; Mulder, JG; Sleijfer, DT. Lactobacillus septicemia, an unusual complication during the treatment of metastatic choriocarcinoma. *Gynecol Oncol.*, 1991 Jan, 40(1), 87-9. PubMed PMID: 1899232. Epub 1991/01/01. eng.

[53] Cornely, OA; Hiddemann, W; Link, H; Maschmeyer, G; Glass, B; Buchheidt, D; et al. Interventional antimicrobial Therapy in Febrile Neutropenic patients (PEG study II) Acute Leukemias VII In: Hiddemann W, Buchner T, Wormann B, Ritter J, Creutzig U, Keating M, et al., editors. Haematology and Blood Transfusion. Hematology and

Blood Transfusion. Berlin-Heidelberg: Springer Berlin Heidelberg; 1998. p. 1045-9.

[54] Anhalt, JA. Antimicrobial susceptibility testing of aerobic and facultative anaerobic bacteria. In: Washington I, J.A., editor. *Laboratory procedures in Clinical Microbiology.*, New York, NY: Spring-Verlag; 1985. p. 281-313.

[55] Chomarat, M; Espinouse, D. Lactobacillus rhamnosus septicemia in patients with prolonged aplasia receiving ceftazidime-vancomycin. *Eur J Clin Microbiol Infect Dis.*, 1991 Jan, 10(1), 44. PubMed PMID: 2009881. Epub 1991/01/01. eng.

[56] Bourne, KA; Beebe, JL; Lue, YA; Ellner, PD. Bacteremia due to Bifidobacterium, Eubacterium or Lactobacillus; twenty-one cases and review of the literature. *Yale J Biol Med.*, 1978 Sep-Oct, 51(5), 505-12. PubMed PMID: 749356. Pubmed Central PMCID: 2595696. Epub 1978/09/01. eng.

In: Bacteremia
Editor: Jodie P. Williams

ISBN: 978-1-63117-290-8

Chapter III

Bacteremia of Oral Origin: Efficacy of Antibiotics and Antiseptics for the Prevention of Potential Complications

***V. Quintas*[1], *I. Prada-López*[1], *N. Donos*[2], *M. Álvarez-Fernández*[3] and *I. Tomás*[1,*]**

[1]Oral Sciences Research Group, School of Medicine and Dentistry, University of Santiago de Compostela, Galicia, Spain

[2]Department of Periodontology, Eastman Dental Institute, University College London, London, United Kingdom

[3]Microbiology, CHUVI, Xeral-Cíes Hospital, IBIV, Vigo, Spain

Abstract

Expert Committees have developed antimicrobial protocols for the prevention of potential complications derived from bacteremia of oral origin, such as infective endocarditis. These preventive protocols have subsequently been revised and modified based on the extensive research

* Corresponding author: Dr. Inmaculada Tomás. Oral Sciences Research Group, School of Medicine and Dentistry, University of Santiago de Compostela, Spain. E-mail: inmaculada.tomas@usc.es. TLF: (+34) 981563100-12344.

that has been performed in this field, including studies on the efficacy of antimicrobial prophylaxis in the prevention of bacteremia of oral origin. The aim of this chapter is to provide an overview of existing studies about bacteremia secondary to dental procedures in humans, showing results concerning the efficacy of both antibiotic and antiseptic prophylaxis, as well as presenting which are the most studied active principles, their doses or concentrations, time and route of administration or the application technique.

The prevention of bacteremia of oral origin has mostly focused on the use of antibiotic prophylaxis prior to dental extractions. However, there are important differences with respect to the type and dose of antibiotic used and time of administration. Penicillins have been the most-studied antibiotics for bacteremia prophylaxis both by oral and parenteral routes. The doses and time of administration varied from 1–3 g and 1–2 hours, respectively, for the oral route which has been the most-studied route of administration. Clindamycin, azithromycin and cephalosporin have been posed as alternatives in allergic patients, although fewer studies exist concerning their prophylactic efficacy.

Some Expert Committees have recommended another complementary method for the prevention of bacteremia of oral origin, which is antiseptic prophylaxis. Numerous reports exist concerning the efficacy of antiseptics at preventing bacteremia secondary to dental procedures. However, there are significant methodological differences related to the dental treatment, the type of antiseptic used and its concentration, as well as the application technique of the antiseptic solution (mouthwash, toothbrush and/or irrigation). The mouthwashes, performed individually or in combination with irrigation, have been the most-studied application technique. Regarding the antiseptic protocol, chlorhexidine has been the most-tested antimicrobial agent, although povidone iodine and essential oils appear to be possible options. However, none of them has been demonstrated to be clearly effective at reducing bacteremia secondary to dental procedures.

Nowadays, the controversies concerning the efficacy of antibiotic prophylaxis and the risk/cost-benefit relationships of antibiotic prophylaxis might justify the convenience of more extensive research on the recommended chlorhexidine regimens and new antiseptic protocols, specifically analysing their effect on the magnitude and duration of bacteremia of oral origin.

In general terms, further evidence-based well-designed research on the efficacy of antimicrobials in the prevention of oral bacteraemic episodes is needed. This is in order to reach a major consensus in the scientific community on the antimicrobial prophylaxis of potential complications, derived from a bacteremia of oral origin.

1. Introduction

The oral cavity is intensely colonised by bacteria. The maximum concentration is found in bacterial plaque, where it is estimated that there are between 10^{11} and 10^{12} microorganisms per gram wet weight [1]. More than 700 bacterial species or phylotypes have been isolated from inside the oral cavity, over 50% of which are not cultivable [2]. As a result, recently developed methods for the specific detection and identification of microorganisms, particularly polymerase chain reaction (PCR) techniques, have renewed interest in this field, as shown by studies performed by several authors [3-7].

In 1999, in a paper published in Science, Costerton et al. showed that 65% of all diseases around the world were produced by biofilms [8]. In 2004, the National Institutes of Health highlighted the major clinical importance of biofilms, affirming that they could be responsible for more than 80% of human body infections. Taking this into account, it must not be forgotten that biofilms develop spontaneously on different oral substrates (teeth, implants, prostheses and oral epithelia) (Figure 1) [9]. A feature that is unique to this oral biofilm, particularly the subgingival plaque, is its close proximity to a highly vascularised milieu (Figure 2). Consequently, any disruption of the natural integrity between the biofilm and the subgingival epithelium barrier, which is at most about 10 cell layers thick [10], places the internal body environment in contact with a highly contaminated ecosystem, resulting in the penetration of microorganisms into the bloodstream [11]. This potential invasion by bacteria might follow a wide variety of dental procedures or manipulations [12].

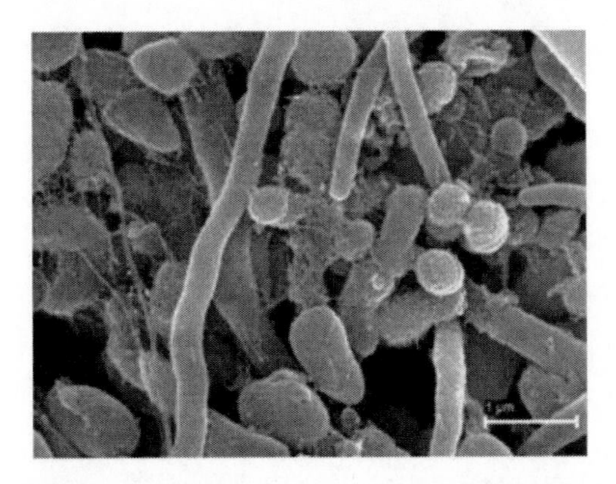

Figure 1. Bacteria present in oral biofilm. Image from a Scanning Electron Microscope (FESEM Ultra Plus, ZEISS, Germany).

Until a few years ago, the detection of a positive post-dental manipulation blood culture was considered to indicate bacteremia of oral origin. However, in 2004, the British Cardiac Society (BCS) and the Royal College of Physicians (RCP) of London established a new concept of bacteremia of oral origin defined as *"bacteremia that is statistically significant with respect to the bacteremia present at baseline"* [13].

In 1885, Osler et al. [14] were the first authors to describe bacteremia secondary to surgery. However, it was not until 1935, that Okell and Elliott [15] first demonstrated the presence of bacteria in the bloodstream after a dental manipulation. Two years later, Burket and Burn [16] injected *Serratia marcescens* into the gingival sulcus of 90 patients and after dental extraction, isolated the bacterium in 20% of the blood cultures, confirming that microorganisms of the oral flora could reach the general circulation during a dental extraction.

In 1945, Bender and Pressman [17] stated that the practice of dental extractions represented the portal of entry of bacteria into the bloodstream through the disruption of blood vessels present in the gingival sulcus and that this was due to the pumping effect caused by such manipulation. Since then, tooth extractions have been considered the dental procedure most frequently associated with bacteremia [18] and during the last 50 years, numerous studies have linked dental treatment with bacteremia and many case reports have linked dental procedures and infective endocarditis (IE) [4, 6, 18-26], but no absolute cause-and-effect relationship has been established [27].

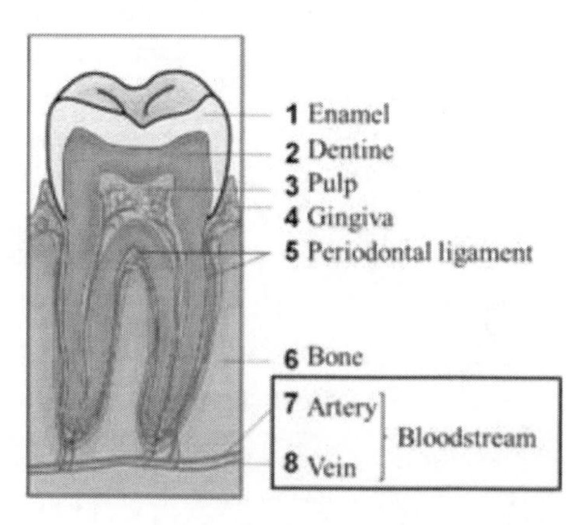

Figure 2. Scheme of a tooth and the surrounding tissues. Notice the high vascularisation, especially in the gingival, periodontal space and periapical region.

The prevalence of bacteremia secondary to dental manipulation is related to the type of dental treatment performed. It varies vastly from one study to another, due to variables such as the time at which the post-extraction blood sample is taken, which in some cases alters the final result. The time-range for samples taken during the procedure [28], is 30 seconds [29, 30], 2 minutes [31] or later. Among other factors, this explains why the prevalence of post-extraction bacteremia varies from 39% [29] to 100% [31]. The percentage prevalence of bacteremia after different dental procedures is shown in Table 1.

The presence of bacteria in the bloodstream has been traditionally assessed by blood cultures. This can cause problems, as previously stated, because there are many species present in the oral cavity that are not culturable [2], which will therefore not appear in the blood. Reports published before the 1960s might also underestimate the incidence of transient bacteremia, since no refined anaerobic culture technique was available [32]. Recently, new methods for the isolation of microorganisms from the bloodstream, which combine anaerobic culture techniques and mainly PCR followed by pyrosequencing, have opened a new area in this field [7, 28].

Table 1. Prevalence of bacteremia following surgical and non-surgical dental manipulations

SURGICAL PROCEDURES	PREVALENCE OF BACTEREMIA Median (range)
Dental extraction	Children: 52% (39–76%) Adults: 75% (39–100%)
Third molar extraction	50% (10–62%)
Periodontal surgery	40% (30–60%)
Maxillofacial surgery techniques	18% (0–58%)
Titanium plaques removal	8% (0–20%)
Incision and drainage of abscess	12%
Stitches removal	10% (5–16%)
Implants surgery	7% (3–23%)
NON-SURGICAL PROCEDURES	PREVALENCE OF BACTEREMIA Median (range)
Conservative procedures	22% (4–66%)
Orthodontic procedures	22% (3–57%)
Endodontic procedures	15% (0–42%)
Local anaesthetic techniques	73% (16–97%)
Scaling and root planing	43% (8–90%)

In 1997, the American Health Association (AHA) stated that: "Bacteremia of oral origin is of a transitory nature as it does not usually persist for more than 15 minutes after completion of the dental procedure" [33]. Due to its transient nature [11], under normal conditions, bacteria move from the bloodstream to the tissues and are rapidly eliminated by the immune system [34, 35]. Although the percentages shown in the Table 1 are relatively low in most cases, it must not be forgotten that the presence of microorganisms in the bloodstream can cause tremendous complications to some susceptible individuals. In addition, it has been suggested that bacteremia might be responsible for some infective-related diseases, such as distant abscesses or failed joint prostheses. Those who suffer from previous cardiac damage [36], malformation [37] or artificial valvular prostheses, will be more exposed than others to bacteria, causing serious damage or even death. Due to this, bacteremia has been traditionally linked to IE [38] which is defined as "an infection of the endocardial surface of the heart, which may include one or more heart valves, the mural endocardium, or a septal defect" (Medscape).

In the literature, the percentage of IE associated with dental manipulation ranges from 4% [39] to 64% [40]. Although patient fatalities associated with such alterations have decreased significantly, the mortality rate remains in the range of 5–11% [11]. Apart from IE, another important complication has been discovered in recent years; the influence of bacteremia in the progression of the atherosclerosis, and consequently, in ischemic diseases (Figure 3) [41, 42].

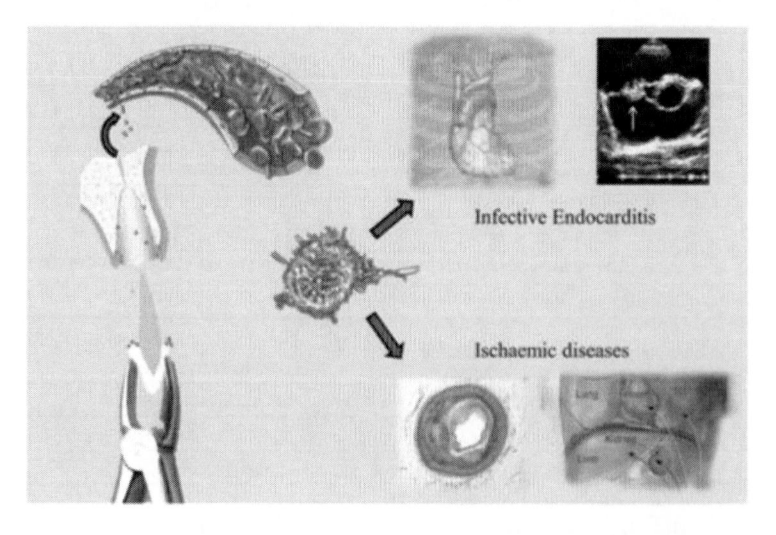

Figure 3. Route of the dissemination of bacteria after a dental extraction and possible complications.

2. Prevention of Potential Complications

As has been previously stated, bacteremia can lead to major complications, with significant morbidity and eventually, mortality [43, 44]. One of the major worries concerning bacteremia of oral origin is the potential IE that can follow a dental procedure, mostly in susceptible patients. It is for this reason, that since the AHA published its first protocol for the prevention of IE associated with dental procedures in 1955, [45] many Expert Committees in different countries have drawn up different prophylactic regimens that have been periodically revised and modified based on: epidemiological and clinical studies, studies of the prevalence of bacteremia secondary to dental procedures, studies on the efficacy of antibiotic prophylaxis (ABP) and antiseptic prophylaxis (ASP), the pharmacokinetics of ABP, the antimicrobial susceptibility of the isolates identified in post-dental manipulation blood cultures, and animal experimentation.

3. Antibiotic Prophylaxis

3.1. Expert Committees Prophylactic Protocols

Controversy concerning efficacy and safety issues with ABP has existed for more than 30 years, and current scientific evidence suggests that dental procedures play a minor role in cases of IE [4, 46]. There is an increasing awareness among experts in this field, of a lack of evidence in general to support the ABP. As a result, since the 1955 AHA guidelines, there has been a progressive reduction in the patient populations with cardiac conditions who warrant ABP, and in the dental procedures considered “at risk”, as well as the dose and duration of ABP [47]. Many IE prophylaxis protocols exist from all over the world. For practical reasons, in this chapter we focus basically on 3 of the most well-known protocols: from the AHA, the British Society for Antimicrobial Chemotherapy (BSAC) and the National Institute for Health and Clinical Excellence (NICE), making references to others in some cases. Although these protocols coincide in some aspects, for example, that there is not enough literature evidence on this issue, they do not agree in some other important questions relating to dental procedures. This is because to date, there has not been a prospective, randomised, placebo-controlled trial aimed at evaluating the efficacy and safety of ABP in IE prevention [48]. Therefore, every professional who relies on a particular protocol might provide a prophylaxis that nearby practitioners do not recommend. The large differences between IE protocols, in addition to the many reviews that are being published, cause, in some cases, confusion among dentists (as well as physicians), which has been demonstrated in published studies concerning the knowledge of professionals with regard to the IE prophylaxis protocols recommended by Expert Committees [48, 49].

In 2006, the BSAC [50] reviewed the current guidelines at that time on IE prophylaxis (those from the AHA [33] and the European Society of Cardiology, ESC [51]), including the published evidence linking a wide range of procedures with the risk of IE in susceptible individuals, and was the fourth revision since their first IE prophylaxis protocol in 1982 [52], and introduces some changes in their recommendations.

A year later, the AHA published its ninth revision [47] since their first IE prophylactic protocol was published in 1955. In this revision, they greatly reduced the number of people recommended for ABP and redefined dental procedures considered to put these people at risk. These current AHA guidelines focus on 4 groups of cardiac patients at the highest risk of experiencing a "bad outcome" resulting from IE, and they no longer recommended ABP for the remaining approximately 90 per cent of patients in the moderate-risk group who before 2007 were recommended to receive ABP [33].

The BCS, which did not agree BSAC protocols from 2006, countered by arranging for the NICE to review matters. As a result, NICE published its own guidelines in 2008 [53]. These were based on systematic reviews of the best available evidence. They stated that both the BSAC [50] and the AHA [47] had recently highlighted the prevalence of bacteremia that was arising from everyday activities such as toothbrushing, the lack of association between episodes of IE and prior interventional procedures, and the lack of efficacy of ABP regimens guidelines. This is one of the reasons why the NICE guidelines have eliminated the use of ABP altogether for all patients with cardiac conditions and for all dental procedures.

The recommendations given by these 3 societies on major questions related to bacteremia and dental procedures have been summarised in Tables 2, 3 and 4. They also provide an idea of the differences that exist between these 3 protocols.

Table 2. Cardiac conditions in which according to AHA, BSAC and NICE should be given antibiotic prophylaxis

PATIENTS WITH HISTORY OF THE FOLLOWING SITUATIONS SHOULD BE GIVEN ANTIBIOTIC PROPHYLAXIS		
AHA	BSAC	NICE
- Prosthetic cardiac valve - Previous infective endocarditis - Cardiac transplantation recipients who develop cardiac valvulopathy - Congenital heart disease (CHD)	- Cardiac valve replacement surgery - Previous infective endocarditis - Surgically constructed systemic or pulmonary shunt or conduit	None

Table 3. Dental procedures which according to AHA, BSAC and NICE should be preceded by antibiotic prophylaxis

DENTAL PROCEDURES FOR WHICH ANTIBIOTIC PROPHYLAXIS IS RECOMMENDED		
AHA	BSAC	NICE
All dental procedures that involve manipulation of gingival tissue or the periapical region of teeth, or perforation of the oral mucosa	All dental procedures involving dento-gingival manipulation	None

Table 4. Antibiotic prophylaxis regimens recommended by AHA, BSAC and NICE

PROPHYLACTIC REGIMENS. (IM, INTRAMUSCULAR; IV, INTRAVENOUS)			
	AHA	BSAC	NICE
Routine	Amoxicillin 2 g	Amoxicillin 3 g	None
Unable to take oral medication	Ampicillin 2g IM/IV	Amoxicillin 50 mg/kg IM/IV	None
Routine but allergy to penicillin	Clindamycin 600 mg	Clindamycin 600 mg	None
Allergy to penicillins or ampicillins and unable to take oral medication	Clindamycin 600 mg IM/IV	Clindamycin 300 mg IV	None

3.2. Efficacy of Antibiotic Prophylaxis

3.2.1. To Prevent Infective Endocarditis

Despite the continual reviews of the ABP protocols, the incidence of IE of possible oral origin has not decreased in recent decades. Delahaye and De Gevigney [54] suggested various reasons to explain this situation: an increase in the number of patients susceptible to IE and in the practice of "at risk" dental procedures, the lack of compliance with the prophylactic regimes for the prevention of IE by doctors, dentists and patients, and the inefficacy of the prophylactic protocols.

Although it has been demonstrated that antibiotics are effective at preventing IE in experimental animals [55-57], the efficacy of prophylaxis in humans has not been analysed and it is clear that no analysis can occur [58]. Moreover, caution must be observed when extrapolating the results obtained on the efficacy of ABP in experimental models to humans [59], principally due to the different rates of excretion of the antibiotics in animals and humans [60]. For example, the half-life of amoxicillin is of 20 minutes in rats, but varies between 50 and 60 minutes in humans.

According to Durack [61], a retrospective series with more than 6,000 patients with heart disease who received a prophylaxis regime or a placebo before undergoing a dental procedure would be necessary to perform a definitive evaluation of the effectiveness of ABP on the prevalence of IE. For other authors [62], the undertaking of a randomised, controlled trial would require the inclusion of approximately 60,000 patients "at risk" of IE over a period of 2 years.

Some authors have suggested that, even assuming that ABP were effective in 100% of cases, its administration would only prevent a small number of cases of IE [63]. In 1992, van de Meer et al. [64] performed a retrospective analysis of 427 cases of IE diagnosed in Holland, of which 275 cases corresponded to patients classified as "at risk" (197 due to the presence of a heart lesion and 78 with prosthetic valves). Sixty-four (23%) of these patients had undergone a dental procedure requiring prophylaxis in the 180 days prior to the onset of symptoms, although only 17 patients had received a IE prophylaxis regimen. Thirty-one patients (11%) had received dental treatment in the previous 30 days and only 8 of these had received ABP. These findings enabled the authors [64] to conclude that: *"Assuming an incubation period of 180 days, the administration of prophylaxis would have avoided cardiac infection in 47 patients, representing only 17% of the IE diagnosed in patients with heart disease undergoing procedures requiring prophylaxis."*

Strom et al. [65], in 1998, estimated that even with ABP with a 100% efficacy, the incidence of IE would be reduced by only 2 cases/1,000,000 population/year, considering a frequency of 5 cases of IE/100,000 population/year in the general population.

3.2.2. Preventing Bacteremia of Oral Origin

Many studies in the literature address the efficacy of ABP in the prevention of bacteremia secondary to dental procedures. They all reveal important differences with respect to the type of antibiotic used, the dose, the route and the time of administration [20, 21, 25, 66-88] (Tables 5 and 6).

Oral Antibiotic Prophylaxis

This route of administration has been the most common use for ABP [21, 25, 66-75, 81-83, 85, 87].

Shanson et al. [21], in 1978, found that the oral administration of a beta-lactam agent (2 g penicillin V or amoxicillin 1 hour before surgery) significantly reduced the prevalence of positive blood cultures 2 minutes after completing a dental extraction in a group of 120 adults, but found practically no difference in the results obtained with the 2 antibiotics (20% and 25%, respectively, *versus* 70% in the controls). This significant reduction in the number of cases of bacteremia was observed for both, those of streptococcal nature and those caused by obligate anaerobic bacteria [21]. Furthermore, in children undergoing dental treatment under general anaesthetic, Roberts et al. [67] demonstrated the efficacy of a single dose of amoxicillin (50 mg/kg bodyweight) administered orally 2 hours before the intervention, as 38% of the controls presented positive blood cultures 2 minutes after completion of the manipulation *versus* 2% of the children receiving the prophylactic regimen.

In contrast to the above results, Hall et al. [69] did not find that prophylaxis with penicillin V or amoxicillin significantly reduced the prevalence or magnitude of post-extraction bacteremia. The percentage of positive blood cultures obtained in this series during surgery were 95% (0.84 CFU/mL) in the "placebo group", 90% (0.66 CFU/mL) in the "penicillin V group" and 85% (1.08 CFU/mL) in the "amoxicillin group"; and after 10 minutes, were 80% (0.36 CFU/mL), 70% (0.36 CFU/mL) and 60% (0.24 CFU/mL), respectively.

Furthermore, the ABP did not affect the aetiology of the bacteremia, as the predominant microorganisms in the 3 groups were *Streptococcus intermedius*, and the most frequent obligate anaerobic bacteria were *Actinomyces* spp., *Peptostreptococcus* spp. and *Veillonella* spp. [69].

Table 5. Principal studies published on the effect of antibiotic prophylaxis on the prevalence and duration of bacteremia secondary to dental manipulations [21, 25, 66-75, 81-83, 85, 87]

	AUTHOR, YEAR [ref.]	SAMPLE GROUP	DENTAL PROCED.	AGENT	POSOLOGY	PREVALENCE OF BACTEREMIA			
						≤5min	10–15 min	30 min	45min–1h
ORAL	Shanson et al., 1978 [21]	120	Extraction	CONTROL	Ø	70%[1]			
				PEN V	2 g, 1 h bf	20%[1]			
				AMX	2 g, 1 h bf	25%[1]			
	Head et al., 1984 [85]	25	Extraction	PLACEBO	2 g, 1 h bf	84%			
				MTZ	2 g, 1 h bf	52%			
				PEN V	2 g, 1 h bf	20%			
	Josefsson et al., 1985 [70]	51	3rd molar surgery	CONTROL	Ø	55%	30%		
				PEN V	2 g, 1–1.5 h bf	50%	15%		
				ERY	500 mg, 1.5–2.5 h bf	55%	20%		
	Shanson et al., 1985 [66]	82	Extraction	PLACEBO	1.5 g, 1 h bf	43%[2]			
				ERY	1.5 g, 1 h bf	15%[2]			
	Roberts et al., 1987 [67]	94*	Extraction	CONTROL	Ø	38%			
				AMX	50 mg/kg, 2 h bf	2%			
	Sefton et al., 1990 [71]	60	Extraction	PLACEBO	1.5 g, 1–1.5 h bf	65%[2]			
				ERY	1.5 g, 1–1.5 h bf	60%[2]			
				JM	1.5 g, 1–1.5 h bf	70%[2]			
	Göker and Güvener, 1992 [68]	100	3rd molar surgery	PLACEBO	1 h bf & 4 days af	44%			28%
				CL	150 mg, 1h bf & af[3]	40%			24%
				OFX	200 mg, 1h bf & af[3]	40%			24%
				SUTN	375 mg, 1h bf & af[3]	36%			24%
	Hall et al., 1993 [69]	60	Extraction	PLACEBO	1 h bf	95%	80%		
				PEN V	2 g, 1 h bf	90%	70%		
				AMX	3 g, 1 h bf	85%	60%		
	Aitken et al., 1995 [72]	40	Extraction	ERY	1.5 g, 1–1.5 h bf	60%[2]			
				CL	600 mg, 1 h bf	40%[2]			
	Hall et al., 1996 [73]	38	Extraction	ERY	1 g, 1.5 h bf	79%	58%		
				CL	600 mg, 1.5 h bf	84%	53%		
	Hall et al., 1996 [87]	39	Extraction	PLACEBO	1g, 1 h bf	85%	47%		
				CCL	1g, 1 h bf	79%	53%		
	Lockhart et al., 2004 [75]	100*	Extraction	PLACEBO	50 mg/kg, 1 h bf	76%	18%	16%	14%
				AMX	50 mg/kg, 1 h bf	15%	2%	0%	0%

	AUTHOR, YEAR [ref.]	SAMPLE GROUP	DENTAL PROCED.	AGENT	POSOLOGY	PREVALENCE OF BACTEREMIA			
						≤5min	10–15 min	30 min	45min–1h
ORAL	Diz Dios et al., 2006 [25]	221	Extraction	CONTROL	Ø	96%	64%		20%
				AMX	2 g, 1 h bf	46%	11%		4%
				CL	600 mg, 1 h bf	85%	70%		22%
				MOX	400 mg, 1 h bf	57%	24%		7%
	Brennan et al., 2007 [89]	100*	Restoration Pulp therapy Cleaning	PLACEBO	50 mg/kg, 1 h bf	20%	16%		
				AMX		6%	0%		
	Lockhart et al., 2008 [4]	192	Extraction	PLACEBO	2 g, 1 h bf	58%	10%	6%	5%
				AMX		33%	1%	1%	0%
	Morozumi et al., 2010 [81]	20	Scaling and root planing	CONTROL	Ø	90%			
				AZM	500 mg/day, 3 days bf	20%			
	Maharaj et al., 2012 [82]	160	Extraction	CONTROL	Ø	35%			
				AMX	3 g, 1 h bf	7.5%			
				CL	600 mg, 1 h bf	20%			
	Duvall et al., 2013 [83]	20	3rd molar surgery	PLACEBO	2 g, 1 h bf	50%			
				AMX		40%			

AMX = amoxicillin; CCL = cefaclor; CL = clindamycin; ERY = erythromycin; JM = josamycin; MOX = moxifloxacin; MTZ = metronidazole; OFX = ofloxacin; PEN = penicillin; SUTN = sultamicillin.

ORAL = oral administration; PROCED. = procedure; h = hours; mg = milligram; g = gram; kg = kilogram; af = after dental manipulation; bf = before dental manipulation.

* Sample group composed by children.

1 – The culture under aerobic and anaerobic conditions was only performed in 20 subjects in each group.

2 – Percentage of positive blood cultures of a streptococcal nature.

3 – This dose was administered every 6 hours for 4 days.

Recent studies have confirmed the efficacy of amoxicillin in the prevention of bacteremia following dental manipulation. Vergis et al. [74] found a reduction of almost 80% in the prevalence of post-extraction bacteremia after administering prophylaxis with 3 g of amoxicillin. In 2004, Lockhart et al. [75] demonstrated that a dose of 50 mg/kg bodyweight of amoxicillin in children significantly reduced the prevalence of bacteremia secondary to nasal intubation (from 18% to 4%), restorative dental treatment and professional hygiene (from 20% to 6%), and dental extractions (from 76% to 15%). These authors [75] also tested the effect of the prophylactic regimen on the duration of post-dental manipulation bacteremia; 45 minutes after completion of the treatment, the percentage of positive blood cultures was 14% in the "placebo group" *versus* 0% in the "amoxicillin group".

With respect to orally administered antibiotics with bacteriostatic activity, Josefsson et al. [70], in 1985, compared the effect of a dose of 500 mg of erythromycin (administered 1.5–2.5 hours before the intervention) with that of 2 g of penicillin V (administered 1–1.5 hours before the intervention) on the prevalence of bacteremia secondary to the removal of impacted or partially erupted mandibular third molars. No differences in the prevalence of bacteremia between the different patient groups were observed during the manipulation, although the concentration of bacteria in the blood cultures was significantly lower in the patients receiving ABP than in the controls. However, the percentage of positive blood cultures 10 minutes after completion of the manipulation was lower in the patients receiving prophylaxis than in the controls [70]. In the same year, Shanson et al. [66] studied the prevalence of post-extraction bacteremia in a group of 82 healthy adults: 40 of them received prophylaxis with erythromycin stearate (1.5 g) and the remaining 42 received a placebo; both substances were administered orally 1 hour before the dental manipulation. The results of this series showed that erythromycin significantly reduced the frequency of positive post-extraction blood cultures of a streptococcal nature (from 43% to 15%) [66].

Other authors, at the beginning of the 1990s, compared the effect of an oral dose of 1.5 g of erythromycin with that of 1.5 g of josamycin, both administered 1–1.5 hours before the manipulation, on the prevalence of post-extraction bacteremia [71]. In contrast to the findings in previous studies [66], and based on the percentages of positive blood cultures detected (60% and 70% in the "erythromycin group" and "josamycin group", respectively, *versus* 65% in the "placebo group"), these authors [71] stated that none of these macrolides significantly affected the frequency of blood cultures due to *Streptococcus* spp..

In 1995, Aitken et al. [72] evaluated the prophylactic effect of 2 oral prophylactic regimens: 600 mg clindamycin *versus* 1.5 g erythromycin. They observed that clindamycin was more active than erythromycin as the prevalence of post-extraction streptococcal bacteremia after the administration of either drug was 40% and 60%, respectively. One year later, Hall et al. [73] performed a similar study, but did not observe a significant difference in the percentage of positive blood cultures or in the concentration of the bacterial isolates during the dental extraction or 10 minutes after completing the surgical procedure. The prevalence of bacteremia during the dental extraction was 79% (2.05 CFU/mL) in the "erythromycin group" and 84% (0.72

CFU/mL) in the "clindamycin group" and after 10 minutes, was 58% (0.60 CFU/mL) and 53% (0.30 CFU/mL), respectively. Although the number of bacteremia of streptococcal aetiology was not affected by the type of antibiotic administered, the proportion of those produced by obligate anaerobic bacteria was reduced to half in the patients receiving clindamycin compared to those receiving erythromycin [73]. Göker and Güvener [68] found a 44% rate of bacteremia secondary to the removal of horizontally impacted mandibular third molars in a "control group" *versus* 40% in the "clindamycin group". These authors also observed no effect of clindamycin on the prevalence of post-extraction bacteremia 1 hour after completing the manipulation, which was 28% in the "placebo group" and 24% in the "clindamycin group". They also measured the existing bacteremia 24 hours after the dental extractions and found that it was still present (8%) in the "placebo group" and was absent in the other antibiotic groups.

In 2006, Diz Dios et al. [25] compared the effect of a single oral dose of 3 different antibiotics (400 mg moxifloxacin, 2 g amoxicillin and 600 mg clindamycin) administered 1 hour before the start of dental extraction, on the prevention of post-extraction bacteremia in 221 adults patients. The results showed that the moxifloxacin and the amoxicillin prophylactic regimens were effective and significantly reduced the prevalence (at 30 seconds) and duration (at 15 minutes and 1 hour) of positive blood cultures secondary to dental extractions in comparison with the percentage observed in the controls (57%, 24% and 7%, respectively, in the "moxifloxacin group" and 46%, 11% and 4% in the "amoxicillin group" *versus* 96%, 64% and 20%, respectively, in the "control group"). However, the "clindamycin group" showed a higher prevalence and duration of bacteremia after dental extraction than the other antibiotics (85%, 70% and 22% after 30 seconds, 15 minutes and 1 hour, respectively). A year later, in 2007, Brennan et al. [89] tested the effect of a single AHA recommended dose (50 mg/kg) of amoxicillin on the prevention of bacteremia secondary to non-surgical procedures (dental restorations, pulp therapy and tooth-cleaning). A sample of 100 children was randomly divided into a "placebo group" and an "amoxicillin group". All the subjects were under general anaesthesia because of the extension of the treatment and/or their age. Immediately after the end of the treatments, bacteremia was found in 6% and 20% of the amoxicillin and placebo groups, respectively. After 10 minutes, the presence of bacteria was no longer found in the "amoxicillin group" samples, whereas 16% of subjects from the "placebo group" had positive blood cultures. In 2008, following this same methodology, Lockhart et al. [4] conducted a study to assess the efficacy of amoxicillin to reduce the bacteremia after a dental extraction in 192 adult subjects. In the "amoxicillin group", 33% had positive blood cultures 5 minutes after starting the procedure, which was lower than that in the placebo group (58%). Twenty minutes after the dental extraction(s) the results were 1% and 10%, respectively. After 1 hour, no bacteria were found in the "amoxicillin group" whereas 5% of subjects in the "placebo group" still showed positive cultures.

Parenteral Antibiotic Prophylaxis

With regard to parenteral ABP, there are also some published studies [20, 76-80, 86, 88]. Starting in 1968, Elliott and Dunbar [20] demonstrated that prophylaxis with penicillin G administered intramuscularly was more effective for the prevention of post-extraction bacteremia in children aged between 2 and 13 years (8% *versus* 55% in the controls) than the administration of 3 oral doses of 125–250 mg of penicillin (36% *versus* 55% in the controls). In 1982, Baltch et al. [80] investigated the efficacy of prophylaxis with intravenous penicillin G (2 million IU by intravenous infusion over 30–40 minutes, starting the surgical procedure 15 minutes after the completion of the infusion) and that of orally administered penicillin G (500 mg-1 g 30 minutes before the procedure) in patients undergoing dental extractions under general or local anaesthesia. In contrast to the results published previously by Elliott and Dunbar [20], the prevalence of bacteremia 30 minutes after completion of the extractions was similar in the patients receiving intravenous and oral prophylaxis (12% and 14%, respectively), and lower than that observed in patients without ABP undergoing dental extractions under local anaesthesia (27%). The percentages of post-extraction blood cultures in which *Streptococcus* spp. were isolated and of the cultures with polymicrobial aetiology were lower in patients receiving prophylaxis with penicillin (intravenous or oral) compared to the controls. This same research group [79] evaluated the prevalence of bacteremia secondary to scaling with ultrasound in 56 patients with periodontal disease: 28 presented cardiopathies and received 2 million IU of penicillin G 45 minutes to 1 hour before treatment and the remaining 28 were healthy subjects who received no ABP. In this series, the prophylaxis resulted in significant differences in the percentage of positive blood cultures obtained 5 minutes after completion of the manipulation (61% falling to 11%) and in the polymicrobial blood cultures (43% falling to 7%). However, these differences were much more discrete 30 minutes after completion of the procedure, due to the marked fall in the prevalence of bacteremia observed in the controls [79].

Table 6. Principal studies published on the effect of parenteral and topical antibiotic prophylaxis on the prevalence and duration of bacteremia secondary to dental manipulations [20, 76-80, 86, 88]

	AUTHOR, YEAR [ref.]	SAMPLE GROUP	DENTAL PROCED.	AGENT	POSOLOGY	PREVALENCE OF BACTEREMIA		
						≤5min	10–15min	30min
PARENTERAL	Elliott and Dunbar, 1968 [20]	173*	Extraction	CONTROL	Ø	55%		
				PEN V	ORAL 125-250 mg, 3 times 1day bf	36%		
				PEN G	IM 500,000 IU, 30 min–1 h bf	8%		
	Baltch et al., 1982 [80]	62	Extraction	CONTROL	Ø	59%[1]		27%[1]
				PEN G	ORAL 500 mg-1 g, 30 min bf	47%		14%
				PEN G	IV 2 million IU, 45–55 min bf	34%		12%
	Baltch et al., 1982 [79]	56	Scaling	CONTROL	Ø	61%		25%
				PEN G	IV 2 million IU, 45 min–1 h bf	11%		15%
	Hess et al., 1983 [76]	82*	Extraction	PEN G	IM 550,000 or 1.2 million IU, 45 min bf[2]	21%		
	Shanson et al., 1987 [86]	120	Extraction	CONTROL	Ø	32%		
				TEIC	IV 400 mg, bf	2%		
				AMX	IM 1 g, bf	25%		
	Kaneko et al., 1995 [77]	26	Extraction	VCM	IV 1 g, 1 h bf	38%		
	Wahlmann et al., 1999 [88]	59	Extraction	CONTROL	Ø		79%	69%
				CFX	IV 1.5 g, 10 min bf		23%	20%
	Roberts and Hozel, 2002 [78]	77*	Extraction	AMP	IV 627 ± 259 mg, immed bf	17%		
				TEIC + AMK	IV 6 mg/kg + 15 mg/kg, immed bf	22%		
TOPICAL	Bartlett and Howell, 1973 [84]	84	Scaling or Extraction	PLACEBO	3-4 mg, 4 days bf	47%[3] 94%[4]		
				VCM		25%[3] 69%[4]		
	Vergis et al., 2001 [74]	36	Extraction	CONTROL	Ø	89%		
				AMX	ORAL 3 g, 1–2 h bf	10%		
				AMX	TOPICAL 3 g, 1–2 h bf	60%		

AMK = amikacin; AMP = ampicillin; CFX= cefuroxime; PEN = penicillin; TEIC = teicoplanin; VCM = vancomycin. (Continued on next page).

ORAL= oral administration; PARENTERAL = parenteral administration; TOPICAL = topical administration; PROCED. = procedure; IM = intramuscular administration; IV = intravenous administration; IU = international units; min = minutes; h = hours; mg = milligram; g = gram; kg = kilogram; immed = immediately; bf = before dental manipulation.

* Sample group composed by children.

[1] Prevalence of bacteremia in controls undergoing dental extractions under local anaesthesia.

[2] Doses administered to children under and over 6 years of age, respectively.

[3] After scaling treatment.

[4] After dental extraction treatment.

In 1983, Hess et al. [76] detected a 21% rate of positive post-extraction blood cultures in children with heart disease who had received prophylaxis with intramuscular penicillin G. Almost 2 decades later, Roberts and Hozel [78] analysed the effect of various intravenous prophylactic regimens on the prevalence of post-extraction bacteremia in children with congenital heart defects undergoing dental treatment under general anaesthesia. The most frequently used protocols were ampicillin (mean dose 627 mg) and teicoplanin in combination with amikacin (6 mg/kg bodyweight and 15 mg/kg bodyweight, respectively). Similar percentages of positive blood cultures were found (17% and 22%, respectively); these rates were significantly lower than those reported previously by the same research group in children who did not receive ABP [78].

In contrast, in 1995, Kaneko et al. [77] observed that the intravenous administration of vancomycin was ineffective in the prevention of bacteremia secondary to dental extractions, as 38% of the patients who received this glycopeptide prophylactically presented positive post-manipulation blood cultures.

Antibiotics Which Are Not Recommended by Expert Guidelines

To provide new prophylactic antimicrobial alternatives, some authors have investigated the prevalence of bacteremia following dental manipulations after the administration of antibiotics not included in the IE prophylaxis protocols recommended by the Expert Committees. One of these, by Head et al. [85] in 1984, evaluated the efficacy of 2 g metronidazole orally on the prevention of post-extraction bacteremia caused by obligate anaerobes, and compared the results with those obtained after the oral administration of 2 g penicillin V or a placebo. Although prophylaxis with penicillin V was associated with a lower prevalence of post-extraction bacteremia (20% *versus* 52% in the "metronidazole group" and 84% in the "placebo group"), it is interesting to note that gram-negative obligate anaerobes were isolated in the blood cultures of 4 (16%) patients receiving penicillin G, whereas these microorganisms were not identified in any of the blood cultures from the patients receiving metronidazole [85]. In 1987, Shanson et al. [86] demonstrated that the administration of an intravenous bolus of 400 mg teicoplanin significantly reduced the prevalence of post-extraction bacteremia due to *Streptococcus viridans* (from 32% in the "control group" to 2% in the "teicoplanin group"); its efficacy was also superior to that observed after the intramuscular administration of 1 g amoxicillin from 20 to 30 minutes before anaesthetic induction (25%). In 1999, Wahlmann et al. [88] demonstrated that patients receiving 1.5 g cefuroxime intravenously, presented a significantly lower rate of bacteremia after performing multiple dental extractions, than controls. This finding was observed after 10 minutes (79% and 23%, respectively) and 30 minutes (69% and 20%, respectively) after commencing the surgery. In contrast, Göker and Güvener [68] did not achieve a reduction in the prevalence of post-extraction bacteremia after the oral administration of 200 mg ofloxacin and 375 mg sultamicillin 1 hour before the intervention, although these findings were probably affected by the low doses used. In 1996, Hall et al. [87] found that the oral administration of 1 g cefaclor did not influence the prevalence or magnitude of post-extraction bacteremia caused by *Streptococcus viridans* or obligate anaerobic bacteria (either during the manipulation or 10 minutes later).

Following the initial data provided by Bender and Pressman [90] in 1956, another attractive line of research arose: topically administered ABP (Table 6). In 1973, Bartlett and Howell [84] decided to investigate whether the preoperative topical application of vancomycin (starting 4 days before the dental treatment) would reduce the prevalence of bacteremia after performing scaling or a dental extraction. These authors [84] found a lower percentage of positive post-scaling or post-extraction blood cultures after using topical vancomycin (25% and 69%, respectively) than after the application of a placebo substance (47% and 94%, respectively), although the differences between the groups were not significant, probably due to the small sample size. In 2001, Vergis et al. [74] performed the first evaluation of the effect of topically applied amoxicillin on the prevalence of post-extraction bacteremia. The study group was formed of 10 controls and 15 patients who performed a double mouthwash with amoxicillin for 1–2 minutes. Although amoxicillin reduced the percentage of post-extraction bacteremia compared to the controls

(60% *versus* 89%), the small sample size did not allow statistical significance between the groups to be established. According to these authors [74], the efficacy of topical amoxicillin on the reduction of the prevalence of post-extraction bacteremia could be increased by increasing the frequency and duration of the mouthwashes, or even performing several applications during the dental procedure.

3.2.3. New Controversies

Antibiotic of Choice

It is known that the onset of IE of oral origin involves the obligatory development of a previous bacteremia [91]. Some authors continue to attribute a greater importance to the role of post-dental manipulation bacteremia in the development of IE due to its duration, intensity and involvement in a possible new pathogenesis model. More than half the studies published on ABP and post-dental manipulation bacteremia have investigated the efficacy of the prophylactic administration of penicillins [20, 25, 66, 67, 69, 71, 74-76, 78-80, 82, 83] (Figure 4). However, there are fewer studies on the effect of prophylactic administration of other recommended antibiotics (clindamycin, azithromycin and the cephalosporins) (Figure 4) on the prevention of post-dental manipulation bacteremia [68, 72, 73, 81, 88], and the results do not confirm the efficacy of these antibiotics.

The activity of an antibiotic administered for prophylactic purposes against a bacterial inoculum that reaches the general circulation depends on several factors, including the sensitivity profile of the microorganisms responsible for the bacteremia. To date, most of the studies on the prevalence of post-dental manipulation bacteremia have confirmed that most of the bacteria isolated in the blood cultures are sensitive to the antibiotics most frequently recommended in the prophylaxis protocols of the Expert Committees [21, 66, 69, 71-73, 87, 92, 93]. However, increasing resistance to beta-lactams, macrolides and lincosamides has been found in bacteria isolated from the oral flora [94] and this might restrict their use for IE prophylaxis. Other antibiotics, such as the fluoroquinolones, have been shown to be successful in bacteremia prophylaxis following dental extractions [25].

It has been shown that the inefficacy of some ABP regimens for the prevention of post-dental manipulation bacteremia does not necessarily imply that they cannot prevent the development of IE [55-57]. However, more scientific evidence of the effect of ABP on the prevalence, duration and magnitude of bacteremia following dental procedures is needed, which analyses the influence of the increasing prevalence of bacterial resistance in the oral ecosystem [95].

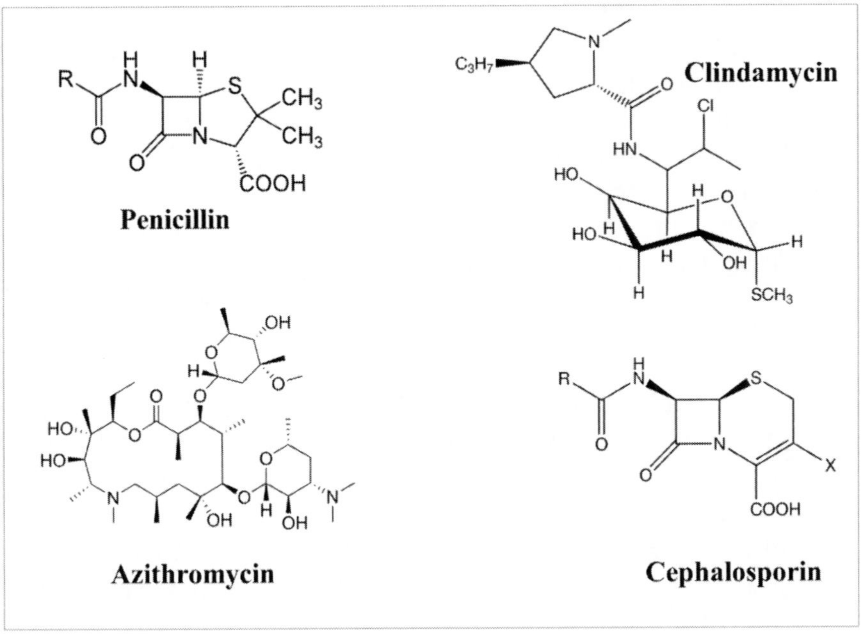

Figure 4. Representations of the chemical formulae of the most commonly used antibiotics for the prevention of bacteremia following dental procedures.

Time of Administration of Antibiotic Prophylaxis

The activity of the antibiotic in the general circulation in the first minutes after the appearance of a bacteraemic episode has been questioned by Hall et al. [69, 73], who considered that the exposure time of the bacteria to the antibiotic was insufficient for it to be able to act. This view is supported by results obtained *in vitro* on the bactericidal activity of various antibiotics against *Streptococcus viridans* [55, 96]. As a consequence, the significant reduction in bacteremia in the initial minutes after completing a dental manipulation reported in some studies is probably not due to the action of the antibiotic in the general circulation. Some authors [72, 97] have suggested that the success of ABP in preventing post-dental manipulation bacteremia might be due to the action of the antibiotic on the bacteria in the oral cavity, before they invade the bloodstream.

In addition to the concentration that the antibiotic reaches in the oral cavity and the antimicrobial sensitivity of oral bacteria, another factor that must be taken into account is the exposure time of the bacteria in the oral cavity to the antibiotic. Some authors [76] have suggested that "*the contact time of the antibiotic with the bacteria in the gingival sulcus might be too short to ensure success of the prophylaxis in the prevention of post-dental manipulation bacteremia*". After a detailed review of the literature, it was interesting to note that in several studies that reported the efficacy of ABP in the prevention of post-dental manipulation bacteremia [25, 67, 75], the antibiotic was administered at least 2 hours before the dental procedure. This might favour the activity of the antibiotic at a "local level" and, therefore, its efficacy in the prevention of bacteremia following dental manipulations.

Assuming this possible mechanism of action of ABP at a dento-alveolar level proposed by some authors [72, 97], the recommended time of administration of oral ABP can be questioned. An increase in the time of contact between the bacteria and the antibiotic in the oral cavity might decrease the prevalence of post-dental manipulation bacteremia, and the reduction in the inoculum size would favour a more rapid elimination of the remaining bacteria from the blood stream by the immune system.

Route of Administration of the Antibiotic Prophylaxis

The BCS and RCP of London [13] published intravenous regimens in 2004, for dental procedures performed under general anaesthesia and for patients with prosthetic heart valves and/or previous episodes of IE. Longman et al. [98] pointed out the "unnecessary use of intravenous prophylaxis for certain risk groups", an affirmation that was corroborated in the last AHA guidelines [47], where intravenous prophylaxis is reserved for patients who cannot take oral medication. This has also been stated in the latest BSAC guidelines [50].

The efficacy of intravenous antibiotics for the prevention of post-dental manipulation bacteremia [79, 80] is similar to that found in studies in which the ABP was administered orally [21, 67, 74, 75]. The mechanism of action of ABP at a dento-alveolar level proposed by some authors [72, 97] might be one possible explanation. Although the intravenous route probably provides higher concentrations of the antibiotic in the oral cavity at the time of the manipulation than oral administration, it has been shown that the oral administration of therapeutic doses of amoxicillin and clindamycin gives rise to high antibiotic concentrations in the gingival fluid (3–4 mg/L and 1–2 mg/L, respectively) [99].

Although the intravenous route provides a higher serum antibiotic concentration at the time of the manipulation than oral administration [67], several authors have demonstrated that amoxicillin and clindamycin taken orally, provides a high serum concentration in the first and second hours after ingestion (15 and 25 mg/L and 4.5 and 4.8 mg/L, respectively), with high levels at 4–6 hours (5 mg/L and 2 mg/L, respectively) and detectable levels still present after 9–10 hours (0.7 mg/L and 0.2 mg/L, respectively). Taking into account that bacterial growth initiates significantly 4 hours after the onset of bacteremia [100], Fluckiger et al. [101] and Dall et al. [57] stated that the prolonged presence of amoxicillin and clindamycin in the bloodstream led to the activation of other defence mechanisms [101].

The low compliance with intravenous guidelines by both patients and practitioners is clear. Consequently, it might be important to perform further studies on the efficacy of intravenous prophylaxis in the prevention of post-dental manipulation bacteremia and experimental IE in comparison with oral prophylaxis.

4. Antiseptic Prophylaxis

4.1. Expert Committee Prophylactic Protocols

Although traditionally, the prophylaxis of bacteremia has been intimately associated with the prescription of an antibiotic prior to the dental manipulation, and has been extensively discussed by most Expert Committees as we have previously stated, there is another type of complementary prophylaxis prior to a dental manipulation that should be taken into account, namely, antiseptic prophylaxis (ASP).

The issue whether antiseptics should be recommended as a complementary measure to ABP has been controversial. Evidence of this previous and current controversy is the fact that in 1997 [33], the AHA recommended the use of antiseptic mouthwashes (containing chlorhexidine or povidone iodine) before certain dental manipulations, but on its latest recommendations [47] and due to the contradictory results concerning its efficacy, they have concluded that there is no clear benefit of antiseptic use to reduce the frequency, magnitude and duration of bacteremia associated with a dental procedure.

Meanwhile, NICE guidelines [53] mention that the issue has been discussed and that there is no agreement between the different scientific societies; in fact, they concluded that ASP should not be offered to people undergoing dental procedures as a prophylaxis against IE. In this same way, the ESC made no reference to the use of antiseptics prior to dental manipulations [102].

However, the BCS [13] and the BSAC [50] agreed in their last respective protocols on the use of pre-operative mouthwashes with 10 mL 0.2% chlorhexidine for 1 minute [50], to reduce the incidence and magnitude of odontogenic bacteremia [13].

This lack of consensus on the need for ASP is probably because the efficacy of chlorhexidine and many other mouthwashes in the prevention of bacteremia after dental procedures has still not been definitively established.

4.2. Efficacy of Antiseptic Prophylaxis

The main objective of ASP is to reduce the bacterial load in the oral cavity at the time the dental manipulation begins, with the aim of minimising the risk of developing bacteremia [63, 97]. It has been demonstrated that a single use of a mouthwash with 0.2% chlorhexidine has a strong antimicrobial effect on the salivary flora [103, 104] and on the supragingival bacterial plaque [105, 106].

It has also been suggested that a single use of a chlorhexidine mouthwash significantly reduces the number of *Streptococcus* species in the gingival sulcus [107]. However, some authors have stated that chlorhexidine mouthwashes do not permeate more than 3 mm into the gingival sulcus (pocket) [108], which could limit the efficacy of the ASP with chlorhexidine mouthwashes in the prevention of bacteremia after dental extractions. Some studies have claimed that chlorhexidine is ineffective in the prevention of bacteremia after dental manipulations, because the forceful use of mouthwashes themselves might cause bacteremia [109].

Other oral antiseptics such as essential oils, cetylpyridinium, chloramine-T, lugol solutions or povidone iodine have also been tested for their ability to reduce bacteremia secondary to dental procedures. A review of the literature on this issue is outlined in the next part of this chapter.

4.2.1. Preventing Bacteremia of Oral Origin

Many studies exist in the literature concerning the efficacy of ASP in the prevention of bacteremia secondary to dental procedures and although chlorhexidine has been the most-tested antiseptic, other antiseptics have been also used in some studies.

However, these studies show major methodological differences, such as the type of dental manipulation performed, the technique for applying the antiseptic (rinse and/or irrigation, toothbrushing, timing, etc.), and the formulation and concentration of the rinse used, making it difficult to compare the results obtained from different studies [19, 30, 81-83, 93, 108-125] (Tables 7, 8 and 9).

Table 7. Principal studies published on the effect of antiseptic prophylaxis applied by mouthwash on the prevalence and duration of bacteremia secondary to dental manipulations [19, 30, 82, 83, 108-111, 115, 121-125]

	AUTHOR, YEAR [ref.]	SAMPLE GROUP	DENTAL PROCED.	AGENT	POSOLOGY	PREVALENCE OF BACTEREMIA		
						≤5min	10–15min	45min –1h
MOUTHWASH	Keosian et al., 1956 [111]	201	Extraction	STERILE SALINE	20 mL, 20 s,bf	27%		
				PI	20 mL, 5 times, 20 s, bf	20%		
	Madsen, 1974 [125]	29	Toothbrushing	CONTROL	Ø	31%		
				CHX	0.2%, 10 mL, 1 min, 2 times/day, 1 week bf	21%		
	Lockhart, 1996 [108]	70	Extraction	PLACEBO	2 times, bf	94%		
				CHX	0.2%,10 mL , 2 times, bf	84%		
	Brown et al., 1998 [109]	61	Stitches removal	CONTROL	Ø	15%		
				CHX	0.12%, 2 times, bf	18%		
	Erverdi et al., 2001 [121]	80	Orthodontic bands colocation[1] or removal[2]	CHX	0.2%, 1 min bf	2.5%[1] 2.5%[2]		
	Cherry et al., 2007 [122]	60	Ultrasonic scaling	PLACEBO	2 min bf	33%		
				PI	7.5%, 2 min bf	10%		
	Tomás et al., 2007 [30]	106	Extraction	CONTROL	Ø	96%	64%	20%
				CHX	0.2%, 30 s bf	79%	30%	2%
	Fine et al., 2010 [123]	62	Chewing an apple	CONTROL	Ø	35.5%		
		22		HYDRO-ALCOHOL	5%, 20 mL, 30 s, 2 times/day, 2 weeks bf	35 CFU/mL[3] 30 CFU/mL[4]		
				EO	20 mL, 30 s, 2 times/day, 2 weeks bf	8 CFU/mL[3] 6 CFU/mL[4]		
	Piñeiro et al., 2010 [124]	50	Implants	CONTROL	Ø	7%	3%	
				CHX	0.2%, 10 mL, 1 min, 30 s bf	0%	0%	

Table 7. (Continued)

	AUTHOR, YEAR [ref.]	SAMPLE GROUP	DENTAL PROCED.	AGENT	POSOLOGY	PREVALENCE OF BACTEREMIA		
						≤5min	10–15min	45min–1h
MOUTHWASH	Cortelli et al., 2012 [126]	109	Chewing an apple	PLACEBO	20 mL, 2 times/day, 2 weeks bf	56 CFU/mL[3] 87 CFU/mL[4]		
		34		EO		11 CFU/mL[3] 26 CFU/mL[4]		
	Maharaj et al., 2012 [82]	80	Extraction	CONTROL	Ø	35%		
				CHX	0.2%, 10 mL, 1 min, 1 h bf	40%		
	Tuna et al., 2012 [19]	34	Extraction	STERIL SALINE	1 min bf	40%	30%	
				CHX	0.2%, 15 mL, 1min bf	25%	17%	
				PI	7.5%, 15 mL, 1 min bf	33%	0%	
	Duvall et al., 2013 [83]	20	3rd molar surgery	PLACEBO	15 mL, 1 min, 15 min bf	50%		
				CHX	0.12%, 15 mL, 1 min, 15 min bf	60%		
MW *vs.* OTHER	Sweet et al., 1978 [115]	100	Extraction	CONTROL	Ø	84%		4%
				C-T	MW 1%, 2 times, bf	48%		0%
				C-T	Brushing 1%, bf	48%		0%
				LUGOL	IRR, bf	80%		0%
	Jokinen et al., 1978 [92]	152	Extraction	CONTROL	Operative field isolation	34%		
				PI	MW 1%, 5–10 mL, 1 min, immed bf	55%		
				PI	TOPICAL 10%, 3–5 min, immed bf	32%		
				CHX	TOPICAL 0.5%, 3-5 min, immed bf	13%		

CHX = chlorhexidine; C-T = Chloramine-T; EO = essential oils; PI = povidone iodine. MW = mouthwash antiseptic application; IRR = antiseptic applied with a needle into the periodontal pocket; TOPICAL = painting the surgical area with the antiseptic; PROCED. = procedure; s = seconds; min = minutes; mL = millilitres; immed = immediately; bf = before dental manipulation; "x" times = number of applications; CFU/mL = colony-forming units per millilitre.

[1] After orthodontic band colocation

[2] After orthodontic band removal

[3] Aerobic bacteria

[4] Anaerobic bacteria

Table 8. Principal studies published on the effect of antiseptic prophylaxis applied by irrigation on the prevalence and duration of bacteremia secondary to dental manipulations [93, 117-119]

	AUTHOR, YEAR [ref.]	SAMPLE GROUP	DENTAL PROCED.	AGENT	POSOLOGY	PREVALENCE OF BACTEREMIA		
						≤5min	10–15min	30min
IRRIGATION	MacFarlane et al., 1984 [93]	60	Extraction	STERILE SALINE	2 min, bf	80%		
				CHX	1%, 2 min, bf	25%		
				PI	1%, 2min, bf	40%		
	Lofthus et al., 1991 [117]	30	Scaling and root planing	CONTROL	Ø	30%[2]		
				STERILE WATER	30 min bf	10%[1] 40%[2]		0%[1]
				CHX	0.12%, 30 min bf	50%[1] 20%[2]		10%[1]
	Allison et al., 1993 [118]	24	Ultrasonic scaling	CONTROL	Ø	75%		
				CHX	0.12% bf & during	25%		
	Rahn et al., 1995 [119]	120	Intraligamentous anaesthesia+ Extraction	STERILE WATER	2 min, bf	52% total from 2 min to 6 min		
				CHX	0.2%, 2 min, bf	45% total from 2 min to 6 min		
				PI	10%, 2 min, bf	27% total from 2 min to 6 min		

CHX = chlorhexidine; CPC = cetylpyridinium chloride; PI = povidone iodine.

IRRIGATION = antiseptic applied with a needle into the periodontal pocket; PROCED. = procedure; s = seconds; min = minutes; bf = before dental manipulation; during = during dental manipulation; "x" times = number of applications.

[1] After subgingival irrigation

[2] After scaling and root planing

Chlorhexidine

The first studies on the antimicrobial efficacy of the chlorhexidine were published in the 1970s. Subsequently, chlorhexidine has been the most-tested antiseptic to date in relation to its effect on the prevalence of bacteremia secondary to dental manipulation, although the results in the literature are quite heterogeneous [19, 30, 82, 83, 93, 108, 109, 117, 118, 121, 124, 125, 127].

Table 9. Principal studies published on the effect of antiseptic prophylaxis applied by irrigation, together with mouthwash on the prevalence of bacteremia secondary to dental manipulations [81, 112-114, 116, 120, 127]

	AUTHOR, YEAR [ref.]	SAMPLE GROUP	DENTAL PROCED.	AGENT	POSOLOGY	PREVALENCE OF BACTEREMIA ≤5min
IRRIGATION + MOUTHWASH	Jones et al., 1970 [112]	201	Extraction	CONTROL	Ø	65%
				STERILE SALINE	MW 30 mL, 30 s bf IRR 20 mL	46%
				PHENOL*	MW 1.4%, 30 mL, 30 s bf IRR 20 mL	18%
	Scopp and Orvieto, 1971 [113]	64	Extraction	PLACEBO	MW 0.5%, 2 times IRR 0.5 %	56%
				PI		28%
	Huffman et al., 1974 [114]	25	3rd molar surgery	STERILE SALINE	MW 20 mL, 15 s, 4 times bf	69%
				CPC	MW 20 mL, 15 s, 4 times bf IRR 20 mL, 15 s, during	83%
	Witzenberger et al., 1982 [116]	64	Scaling	CONTROL	Ø	55%
				PI	MW 10%, 15 mL, 1 min IRR 10%, 10 mL, 3 min bf	40%
	Waki et al., 1990 [127]	60	Scaling and root planing	CONTROL	Ø	13%
				CHX	MW 0.04%, daily/3 months bf IRR 0.12%, 2–7 min	18%
				WATER + CHX	MW daily/3 months bf IRR 0.12%, 2-7 min	27%
				WATER	MW daily/3 months bf IRR 2–7 min	15%
	Fine et al., 1996 [120]	18	Scaling and root planing	HYDROALCOHOL	MW 5%, 20mL, 30 s, bf IRR 10 mL, 30 s, bf	54 CFU/mL
				EO	MW 20 mL, 30 s, bf IRR 10 mL, 30 s, bf	6 CFU/mL
	Morozumi et al., 2010 [81]	20	Scaling and root planing	CONTROL	Ø	90%
				EO	MW 20 mL, 20 s, 4 times/day, 1 week bf IRR 100 mL, 10 min, 1 week bf	70%

CHX = chlorhexidine; CPC = cetylpyridinium chloride; EO = essential oils; PI = povidone iodine. * In solution with sodium phenolate, sodium borate, menthol, thymol and glycine. MW = mouthwash antiseptic application; IRR = antiseptic applied with a needle into the periodontal pocket; PROCED. = procedure; s = seconds; min = minutes; mL = millilitres; bf = before dental manipulation; during = during dental manipulation; "x" times = number of applications; CFU/mL = colony-forming units per millilitre.

In 1974, Madsen [125] demonstrated that performing mouthwashes with 0.2% chlorhexidine digluconate twice a day for one week (without any other complementary technique of oral hygiene) did not significantly condition the percentage of streptococcal bacteremia secondary to the toothbrushing, neither did the use of a toothpick, in patients with gingival affectation. Waki et al. [127] investigated irrigation in the home with 0.04% chlorhexidine in a group of 60 subjects in a periodontal maintenance regimen for 3 months and professional irrigation with 0.12% chlorhexidine prior to a manipulation conditioned the prevalence of bacteremia following scaling and root planing. These results contrast with those from a group of individuals who underwent daily water irrigation and professional irrigation with chlorhexidine prior to a manipulation, another group which received only water irrigation exclusively (both the daily and the professional ones) and a further group that did not receive any type of irrigation. According Waki et al. [127], the low prevalence of post-scaling and root-planing bacteremia detected in the patients who underwent periodontal maintenance, led to the absence of significant differences between the 4 studied groups in relation to the percentage of positive blood cultures post-manipulation, which ranged between 13% and 27%.

In 1978, Jokinen [92] investigated the effectiveness of several local prophylaxis methods in a group of 152 patients undergoing dental extractions: rinsing with 1% povidone iodine for 1 minute, isolation of the operative field (saliva ejector altogether with cotton rolls), isolation of the operative field and painting with 10% povidone iodine, and finally, isolation of the operative field and painting with 0.5% chlorhexidine gluconate solution. The lowest percentage of post-extraction blood cultures was obtained following the isolation of the operative field and disinfection with chlorhexidine (13% *versus* 32–55% in the remaining groups). Therefore, the application of this sequence was recommended before any dental manipulation [92].

In 1984, MacFarlane et al. [93] found that the prevalence of post-extraction bacteremia was significantly lower in patients undergoing gingival sulcus irrigation with 1% chlorhexidine or 1% povidone iodine (keeping the antiseptic solution in the mouth for 2 minutes), than in a group that was exclusively irrigated with saline (the percentages of positive blood cultures were 25%, 40% and 80%, respectively), which confirmed the importance of bactericidal activity more than a simple mechanical washing effect.

As other authors did previously [113], these researchers [93] recommended sulcus irrigation with 1% chlorhexidine or 1% povidone iodine, in addition to the ABP.

In 1991, Lofthus et al. [117] evaluated the effect of previous irrigation upon the gingival sulcus with 0.12% chlorhexidine for 20 seconds on the prevalence of bacteremia caused by scaling and root planing; from the 30 patients studied, 9 presented positive post-manipulation blood cultures: 3 were controls (n = 10), 4 were irrigated with sterile water (n = 10) and 2 with chlorhexidine (n = 10). Consequently, these authors [117] concluded that subgingival irrigation with 0.12% chlorhexidine did not reduce the prevalence of bacteremia secondary to scaling and root planing. Conversely, Allison et al. [118] showed that the application of a 0.12% chlorhexidine irrigating solution at the subgingival level before and during the practice of subgingival scaling, with an ultrasonic scaler, reduced the percentage of bacteremia.

In 1995, Rahn et al. [119] investigated whether gingival sulcus irrigation with 10% povidone iodine or 0.2% chlorhexidine (keeping the solution in the mouth for 2 minutes) conditioned the prevalence of bacteremia associated with certain dental procedures (intraligamentary injection or the extraction of a molar); in this study, on a group of 120 subjects, there was a significant reduction in the frequency of post-intraligamentary injection or post-extraction bacteremia after irrigation with povidone iodine (27%), in contrast with results obtained from irrigation with sterile water (52%) and chlorhexidine (45%). Based on these findings, these authors [119] noted that the most effective method of applying an antiseptic, to reduce the prevalence of post-dental manipulation bacteremia, was sulcular irrigation prior to dental treatment. Similar to findings of other researchers [93], they suggested that the reduction in the bacteremia prevalence of dental post-manipulation was due to the bactericidal action of antiseptics more than to the “mechanical washing effect” of irrigation, and they also showed that povidone showed a greater antiseptic activity than chlorhexidine [119]. However, it should be noted that the povidone was used at a concentration 50 times higher than that of chlorhexidine.

In 1996, Lockhart [108] investigated the prevalence and aetiology of post-extraction bacteremia in a group of adults undergoing 2 consecutive “energetic” rinses with 10 mL of 0.2% chlorhexidine hydrochloride, and in another group of patients who rinsed with a placebo solution. Lockhart [108] concluded that previous rinses with chlorhexidine did not exert a significant effect on the prevalence of post-extraction positive blood cultures, which was 84% in the "chlorhexidine group" and was 94% in the "placebo group". To explain these findings, this author [108] noted that performing a rinse with an antiseptic penetrated no more than 3 mm into the gingival sulcus, and therefore did not reach the area where the bacteria entered the bloodstream.

Brown et al. [109] investigated the effect of a single rinse with 0.12% chlorhexidine hydrochloride on the prevalence and intensity of bacteremia secondary to the removal of stitches; the study group consisted of 61 patients who underwent third molar extractions, closing the surgical bed with at least 8 stitches. After 7 days, patients were distributed into a "control group" and another group composed of subjects who performed a chlorhexidine rinse for 1 minute prior to the removal of the stitches. The overall prevalence of bacteremia associated with suture removal was 18% in the "chlorhexidine group" and 15% in the "control group". Brown et al. [109] explained these findings, by arguing that the practice of oral rinses of “active” character might cause bacteremia and the short duration of the rinse (1 minute) prevented the antiseptic from exerting an antibacterial activity.

Erverdi et al. [121] investigated the prevalence of bacteremia associated with the placement and removal of orthodontic bands after performing a rinse with 0.2% chlorhexidine gluconate for 1 minute, and compared the results to those published previously [128, 129]. After the placement of the bands, the percentage of positive blood cultures was 7.5% in controls and 2.5% in the subject undergoing the rinse with chlorhexidine; after removal of the bands, these percentages were 6.6 and 2.5% respectively.

Similarly, Tomás et al. [30] evaluated the occurrence of bacteremia post-extraction, after a rinse with 0.2% chlorhexidine digluconate prior to the dental extraction. The study group comprised 106 patients with mental or behavioural disabilities who underwent dental extractions under general anaesthesia. The sample group was randomly divided into a control and a test group. Prior to the dental procedure, and after the anaesthesia, the mouth of the subjects was filled with 0.2% chlorhexidine for 30 seconds. Blood samples were collected at baseline (before the start of the dental procedure but after the endotracheal intubation), 30 seconds, 15 minutes and 1 hour after the final extraction. The chlorhexidine diminished the prevalence of post-extraction bacteremia after 30 seconds (79% *versus* 96%), 15 minutes (30% *versus* 64%) and 1 hour (2% *versus* 20%). According to the authors, an initial 0.2% chlorhexidine mouthwash should be performed by all patients, to reduce the prevalence and duration of bacteremia secondary to dental extractions.

In 2010, this same group published a study [124] on the efficacy of 0.2% chlorhexidine digluconate in reducing the prevalence of bacteremia secondary to implant placement. The study group consisted of 50 patients undergoing implant placement surgery with a mucoperiosteal flap. Patients were randomly allocated into the test group (20) or the control group (30), which did not receive any type of prophylaxis. Blood samples were taken at baseline, 30 seconds after the placement of the implants and 15 minutes after the flap was completely sutured. After obtaining 2% bacteremia at baseline, there were no positive blood cultures after the 0.2% chlorhexidine mouthwash, with 7% at 30 seconds and 3% at 15 minutes in the control group. Due to the data from the control group, the authors concluded that implant placement with a mucoperiosteal flap did not carry any significant risk of developing a bacteremia. Even though the efficacy of chlorhexidine was not statistically confirmed, they reinforced their recommendation for its use before a dental treatment, to reduce the bacterial load present in the oral cavity.

Recently, Tuna et al. [19] compared the prophylactic effect of 0.2% chlorhexidine and 7.5% povidone iodine in 34 patients who underwent third-molar surgery. All patients were divided into 3 groups; the first 12 patients received a prophylactic mouthwash with 15 mL povidone iodine at 7.5%, the next 12 patients rinsed with 15 mL 0.2% chlorhexidine and 10 patients rinsed with sterile saline (0.9% NaCl). All mouthwashes were performed 1 minute before the start of surgery. The prevalence of bacteremia 1 minute after the extraction was 33%, 25% and 40%, in the povidone iodine, chlorhexidine and control groups, respectively. After 15 minutes of surgery, the prevalence was reduced to 0% in the povidone iodine group, 17% in the chlorhexidine group and 30% in the control group. These results showed that chlorhexidine and povidone iodine had a noticeable prophylactic effect. Although chlorhexidine was more effective than povidone iodine at reducing the prevalence of bacteremia after the first minute, these results differed after 15 minutes of the dental manipulation, when povidone iodine was more effective than chlorhexidine.

Other Oral Antiseptics

One of the first published studies on this issue was that from Keosian et al. [111], who tested the efficacy of 5 mouthwashes in a water solution of iodide (20 mL each for 20 seconds) in the reduction of the prevalence of post-extraction bacteremia, and compared the results with those obtained from rinsing with a saline solution; in this study, a low prevalence of post-extraction bacteremia was recorded (20% of blood cultures were positive in those patients who used the iodide solution *versus* 27% from those who used the saline solution). This reflected that the influence of the "washing effect" inherent to the action of rinsing is greater than the antibacterial activity of the iodide solution itself. In this study, most of the patients with positive post-extraction blood cultures presented local infections (odontogenic abscesses, chronic pulpitis and/or periodontitis), which permitted the authors [111] to suggest that if the traumatized areas were also infected, a greater probability of bacterial dissemination into the bloodstream existed, even after prior iodide mouthwashes.

In contrast to the results of Keosian et al. [111] on the use of iodide mouthwashes, Rise et al. [110] demonstrated in 1969, that performing 3 mouthwashes with buffered monohydrated sodium perborate for 30 seconds reduced the prevalence of bacteremia secondary to periodontal procedures and extractions 15 minutes after dental manipulation; these authors [110] were the first to recommend the routine practice of mouthwashes with buffered monohydrated sodium perborate, prior to any dental manipulation in which ABP was not used.

A year later, Jones et al. [112] investigated whether the combination of a mouthwash and irrigation of the gingival sulcus significantly reduced the prevalence of bacteremia secondary to dental extractions. The study group consisted of 201 patients, who were randomly distributed into 3 groups: a control, a group that used saline and a third group that employed an antiseptic with 1.4% phenol, sodium phenolate, sodium borate, menthol, tymol and glycerine. The reduction in the number of post-extraction positive blood cultures between the patients using saline compared with the controls (46% *versus* 65%), confirmed the "washing effect" produced by the combination of rinsing and irrigation; nevertheless, the significant differences detected among patients using saline compared to those using the antiseptic (46% *versus* 18%), also revealed the bactericidal activity exerted by this agent. To explain the occurrence of positive blood cultures in patients receiving ASP, the authors speculated that the bacteremia was probably less intense. Consequently, Jones et al. [112] recommended rinsing, in combination with gingival sulcus irrigation with an antiseptic phenolated solution prior to dental extraction; for these authors [112], this prior action was not intended to replace the administration of ABP in patients considered "at risk" of IE, but the application of an antiseptic was presumed to provide additional protection against the emergence of post-extraction bacteremia.

In 1974, Huffman et al. [114] evaluated the effect of 4 rinses of cetylpyridinium chloride (20 mL each for 15 seconds) and its posterior application as an irrigant solution during surgery in a group of 25 individuals, in the appearance of bacteremia associated with the extraction of impacted third molars. These authors [114] demonstrated that cetylpyridinium chloride did not significantly reduce the prevalence of post-extraction bacteremia compared to that in subjects who performed mouthwashes with saline. The percentage of positive blood cultures was 83% in the "cetylpyridinium group" and 69% in the "saline group"; a predominance of obligate anaerobic bacteria was clear in both groups (86% and 74%, respectively) [114].

In 1978, Sweet el al. [115] randomly distributed a sample of 100 subjects who were undergoing dental extractions, into 4 groups: controls, patients who performed a double rinse with 1% chloramine-T, patients who brushed with 1% chloramine-T and patients who underwent irrigation with a lugol solution. The results revealed that the double rinse and the toothbrushing with 1% chloramine-T prior to manipulation noticeably reduced the prevalence of bacteremia (48% after the mouthwash or the brushing *versus* 84% in controls); however, irrigation of the gingival sulcus with lugol solution did not alter the prevalence of bacteremia (80% *versus* 84%). Comparing the effects of both antiseptics, the chloramine-T groups presented significantly fewer positive blood cultures than those treated with the lugol solution, showing that differences existed among the bactericidal activity of both antiseptics, independent of the application method; however, no significant differences were observed in the intensity of the bacteremia among the 4 groups of patients. In this same study, the duration of post-extraction bacteremia was also investigated and revealed only 1 control (4%) with a positive blood culture 1 hour after the extraction, resulting in all-negative blood cultures after 6 hours. These authors [115] proposed the systematic topical use of chloramine-T prior to any dental procedure as a complement to ABP in patients "at risk" of IE.

In 1971, Scopp and Orvieto [113] evaluated the effect of 2 mouthwashes together with irrigation of the gingival sulcus with 0.5% povidone iodine in a group of 64 patients, on the prevalence of bacteremia associated with dental extractions. In this study, the appearance of post-extraction bacteremia was significantly conditioned by the previous administration of povidone iodine, since the percentage of positive blood cultures was 28% in patients who used the antiseptic *versus* 56% in those who were supplied with a placebo. To explain these results, the authors [113] demonstrated that povidone iodine produced the complete elimination or a significant reduction in the number of bacteria present in the gingival sulcus in almost 45% of the patients (with the placebo solution, this was only observed in 3% of the patients).

In the early 1980s, Witzenberger et al. [116] evaluated the effect of povidone iodine mouthwash combined with gingival sulcus irrigation with 10% povidone, on the prevalence of bacteremia associated with the performance of subgingival scaling. The study group was formed of 20 patients, each with "control areas" and "experimental areas" (exposed to the ASP); in contrast to previously obtained results [113], the mouthwash and gingival sulcus irrigation did not reduce the prevalence of positive blood cultures 2 minutes after the start of the scaling (25% *versus* 40%), nor immediately after the end of the manipulation (although the percentage decreased from 55% to 40%). Witzenberger et al. [116], agreeing with the findings of other authors [112], suggested that the local application of povidone iodine might not condition the prevalence, but rather the intensity of the bacteremia post-dental manipulation.

More than 2 decades later, in 2007, Cherry et al. [122] investigated whether povidone iodine can effectively prevent bacteremia secondary to ultrasonic scaling. The study group was formed by 60 patients with gingivitis who were divided into 2 groups of 30; one control group that performed a saline rinse and another group that rinsed with 7.5% povidone iodine. Both groups rinsed for 2 minutes prior to the start of the scaling of the teeth from 31 to 35 (FDI). Blood samples were taken 30 seconds after the start of the procedure and 2 minutes after its end. Three out of the 30 subjects from the povidone iodine group showed a lower bacteremia (10%) than the control group, whereas 10 out of the 30 subjects of the saline group (33%) were shown to have bacteremia. According to these data, the authors concluded that performing a rinse with 7.5% povidone iodine significantly reduced the bacteremia produced after ultrasonic scaling and was helpful for the ultrasonic scaling of gingivitis patients "at risk" of IE.

In 1996, Fine et al. [120] investigated the impact of subgingival irrigation with essential oils, together with a posterior mouthwash with this same antiseptic, on the intensity of the bacteremia produced, secondary to subgingival scaling with an ultrasonic scaler in patients with periodontal disease; the study group was composed of 18 patients who had previously presented positive blood cultures after scaling with the ultrasonic scaler. These patients underwent irrigation and performed a mouthwash with essential oils, repeating the process the following week with a 5% hydroalcoholic solution. The results in relation to the intensity of the bacteremia secondary to subgingival scaling with an ultrasonic scaler for 5 minutes were 4.67 CFU/mL of aerobic and 1.61 CFU/mL of anaerobic bacteria with the antiseptic solution *versus* 38.72 and 14.89 CFU/mL, respectively, with the hydroalcoholic solution, which demonstrated that irrigation in combination with mouthwash of essential oils significantly reduced the intensity of post-subgingival scaling bacteremia, and minimised the size of the bacterial inoculum in the oral cavity [120]. In 2010, the group of Fine [123] published a further study to assess the effect of a mouthwash containing essential oils on the reduction of bacteremia, after chewing an apple. A total of 22 patients with gingivitis who had previously presented positive blood cultures after chewing an apple were selected for the study and were randomised into 2 groups. One group performed a mouthwash for 30 seconds with a 5% hydroalcoholic solution twice a day for 2 weeks and the other group did the same with a solution of essential oils. After 2 weeks, they were asked to chew and swallow an apple and the level of bacteria present in their bloodstream was measured. This process was repeated after 1 week of washout and once again after a further 2 weeks, when the participants were given the other mouthwash (either the placebo or the test, depending on what they had received in the first period). After these 3 measurements, the conclusions were that the essential oils reduced the bacteria present in the bloodstream by about 69% both for aerobic and anaerobic bacteria, compared to the initial baseline. However, the hydroalcoholic solution had no effect on this reduction. Cortelli et al. [126] performed a similar clinical trial 2 years later. After 2 weeks, the essential oils group presented 46% and 63% fewer aerobic and anaerobic bacteria, respectively, compared to the baseline. The amount of aerobic bacteria in the "placebo group" was even higher than the baseline. These authors [123, 126] concluded that performing daily mouthwashes with essential oils reduced the levels of bacteria in the bloodstream of patients with gingivitis.

Antibiotic Prophylaxis *vs.* Antiseptic Prophylaxis

To the best of author's knowledge, there have only been 3 published studies that have compared ABP with the ASP [81-83] (Table 10).

In 2010, Morozumi et al. [81] investigated whether irrigation and mouthwash with an essential oil-containing antiseptic and oral administration of azithromycin could influence the level of bacteria present in the bloodstream after a scaling and root planing treatment. The study group was formed of 30 patients who were randomised into 3 different study-groups. The first group received 500 mg azithromycin daily for 3 days before the scaling and root planing treatment. The second group received an initial irrigation with 100 mL essential oils and continued with 4 mouthwashes per day, with 20 mL essential oils, the week before the periodontal treatment. The final group was the control and no prophylaxis was given. The blood samples were taken 6 minutes after the treatment was started. The prevalence of bacteria in the blood cultures was 20% in the "antibiotic group" and 70% in the "antiseptic group" *versus* 90% in the "control group". The authors concluded that although a significant reduction of the incidence of bacteremia was shown in the "azithromycin group", only subgingival bacterial counts significantly decreased in both prophylaxis groups.

Table 10. Principal published studies that compare the efficacy of antibiotic prophylaxis with antiseptic prophylaxis on the prevalence of bacteremia secondary to dental manipulations

	AUTHOR, YEAR [ref.]	SAMPLE GROUP	DENTAL PROCED.	AGENT	POSOLOGY	PREVALENCE OF BACTEREMIA
						≤5min
ABP *vs.* ASP	Morozumi et al., 2010 [81]	30	Scaling and root planing	CONTROL	Ø	90%
				AZM	500 mg/day, 3 days bf	20%
				EO	IRR 100 mL, 10 min, 1 week bf MW, 20 mL, 20 s, 4 times/day, 1 week bf	70%
	Maharaj et al., 2012 [82]	160	Extraction	CONTROL	Ø	35%
				AMX	3 g, 1 h bf	7.5%
				CL	600 mg, 1 h bf	20%
				CHX	MW, 0.2%, 10 mL, 1 min, 2 times, 1 h bf	40%
	Duvall et al., 2013 [83]	30	3rd molar surgery	PLACEBO	2 g, 1 h bf MW, 15 mL, 1 min, 15 min bf	50%
				AMX + PLACEBO		40%
				PLACEBO + CHX	2 g, 1 h bf MW, 0.12%, 15 mL, 1 min, 15 min bf	60%

AMX = amoxicillin; AZM = azithromycin; CHX = chlorhexidine; CL = clindamycin; EO = essential oils. ABP = antibiotic prophylaxis; ASP = antiseptic prophylaxis. MW = mouthwash antiseptic application; IRR = antiseptic applied with a needle into the periodontal pocket; PROCED. = procedure; s = seconds; min = minutes; h = hour; mL = millilitres; bf = before dental manipulation; "x" times = number of applications.

Maharaj et al. [82] published a paper in 2012 in which they compared the effectiveness of amoxicillin, clindamycin and chlorhexidine on reducing bacteremia secondary to dental extractions. The study group was composed of 160 patients who underwent dental extractions. These were randomised into 4 different groups with the same number of patients. One group received 3 g amoxicillin, the second one received 600 mg clindamycin and the third one performed a mouthwash with 10 mL 0.2% chlorhexidine for 1 minute, twice (all procedures were performed 1 hour before the start of the dental extraction). The final group was the control group, which did not receive any type of prophylaxis. The blood samples were taken 3 minutes after the end of the dental extraction. The prevalence of bacteremia after the extraction was 7.5%, 20%, 40% and 35% in the amoxicillin, clindamycin, chlorhexidine and control groups, respectively. In this case, the ASP was not effective in reducing the level of bacteria present in the blood after a dental procedure.

Recently, in 2013, Duvall et al. [83] obtained similar results after studying 30 patients who required the extraction of the 4 third molars. The protocol of the first group (10 patients) was 2 g amoxicillin 1 hour before extraction and a mouthwash with 15 mL placebo solution for 1 minute, 15 minutes before the treatment. The next 10 patients received a placebo capsule 1 hour before and they performed a mouthwash with 15 mL chlorhexidine at 0.12% for 1 minute, 15 minutes before the surgery. The final 10 patients received the placebo capsule, 1 hour before, and a placebo mouthwash, 15 minutes before surgery. The results of positive cultures were 40% after the amoxicillin protocol, 60% after chlorhexidine protocol and 50% in the "placebo group".

4.2.2. New Controversies

Antiseptic of Choice

More than half of the studies published on ASP and post-dental manipulation bacteremia have investigated the efficacy of the prophylactic administration of chlorhexidine (Figure 5).

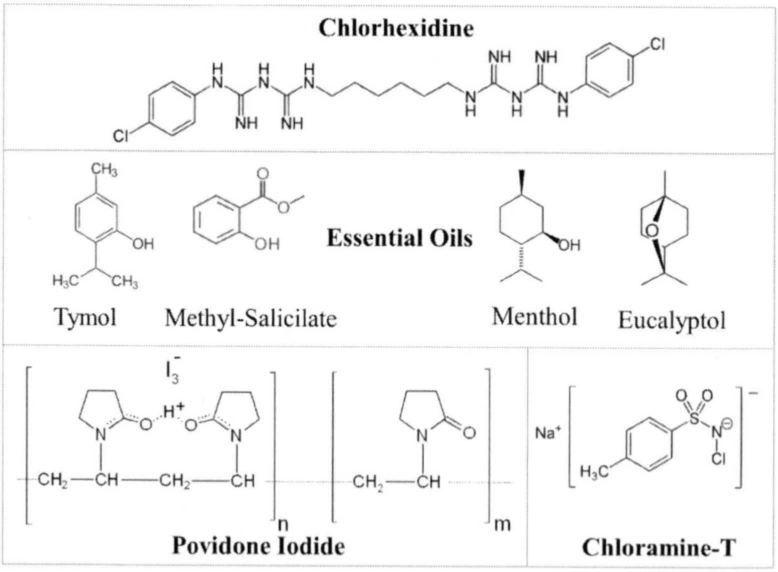

Chlorhexidine

Essential Oils

Tymol Methyl-Salicilate Menthol Eucalyptol

Povidone Iodide

Chloramine-T

Figure 5. Representations of the chemical formulae of the most commonly used antiseptics for the prevention of bacteremia of oral origin.

However, other studies have been published on the efficacy of other antiseptics such as the essential oils, povidone iodine or chloramine-T (Figure 5), among others, with very heterogeneous results.

The Expert Committees that recommend ASP [13, 50], suggest the use of chlorhexidine, and it should be remembered that it is currently the "gold standard" in terms of antisepsis inside the oral cavity [130]. However, some of the reviewed papers [19, 119] showed that chlorhexidine had a small effect on reducing bacteremia secondary to dental procedures that some other antiseptics such as povidone iodine. Although, as usual, other studies exist that obtained the opposite result [92, 93].

Time of Administration of Antiseptic Prophylaxis

Since the objective of a prophylactic mouthwash is to reduce the bacterial load inside the oral cavity prior to a dental procedure, some of the methods followed in some studies are not understandable.

Some studies used antiseptics for a whole week [81, 123] to reduce the bacterial load of the oral cavity, but did not perform any mouthwash prior to the action that caused the bacteremia. In other cases, the ASP was given 1 hour [82] or 15 minutes [83] before the start of the treatment. Appealing to common sense, if we require a drastic reduction in the bacterial load to prevent the entry into the bloodstream of the smallest amount of microbial pathogens, it does not make sense to perform a mouthwash 1 hour prior to a procedure, since at the time of the procedure, the activity of the antiseptic will not be as high as it was at the time the rinse was performed.

However, in most of the studies [19, 30, 92, 110-112, 118, 121, 124], the antiseptic was applied before the start of the dental procedure. However, the importance or the efficacy of the antiseptic application for several days before the manipulation should be studied more deeply, to clarify its possible benefit in comparison to a single application immediately before the start of the dental procedure.

Specific Controversial Issues

It has been also discussed whether the antiseptic should be applied only once or several times [81-83]. This question has been raised, since theoretically, performing a mouthwash twice will kill more bacteria than performing it only once, but it has been suggested that more than one mouthwash might possibly aid the proliferation of resistance among oral pathogenic bacteria [131], which would eventually lead to a major concentration of "bad" bacteria that might enter the bloodstream more easily. In the author's point of view, although this suggestion might make sense, it should not be forgotten that resistance might develop after weeks or months of continuous antiseptic use, but it is hard to believe that resistance could develop after several applications within a short period of time (i.e., one week), in fact, other studies have demonstrated that the repetitive use of an antiseptic does not cause resistance [132].

Another issue that has caused some controversy is that according to some authors, a mouthwash (specifically one containing chlorhexidine) cannot reach more than 3 mm inside the periodontal sulcus [108], which would make it useless because the bacteria that would enter the bloodstream following, for example, a dental extraction, would be those that were nearest to the arteriovenous package, which would be those from the lowest part of the alveolar pocket.

Other authors have obtained worse results with ASP than with performing a saline mouthwash or even with no treatment [82, 109, 117, 127]. They have attributed these results to the fact that a mouthwash will force bacteria inside the periodontal pocket and they will eventually reach the bloodstream [109]. Of course, this theory is not compatible with that published by Lockhart et al. [108], who stated that mouthwash does not reach more than 3 mm inside the periodontal pocket; consequently, it will not force bacteria enter the bloodstream. In fact, a detailed review of the literature has found no rigorously designed studies to support the hypothesis that the forceful use of mouthwashes can cause bacteremia [30]

On the other hand, in 1997, the AHA recommended against the application of antiseptics by means of gingival irrigators [33], probably assuming that subgingival irrigation could favour the passage of oral bacteria into the bloodstream. However, few studies have been published on this subject and their results are contradictory [116, 117].

Some authors have also stated that although ASP is possibly not effective at reducing the prevalence of bacteremia after a dental procedure, it might reduce the magnitude of oral bacteremia [122], which is a lower amount of bacteria in the blood cultures than when ASP was not used. This might indirectly reduce the duration of the episode of bacteremia secondary to a dental manipulation. However, few authors have studied the effect of ASP on the magnitude and duration of post-dental manipulation bacteremia, so that more scientific evidence in this regard is required.

Conclusion

1. Apart from its possible implication in the onset of episodes of infective endocarditis, there has been increasing interest in bacteremia of oral origin in the past 2 decades due to the major role it is considered to play in the progression of atherosclerosis and consequently in the occurrence of chronic diseases. For this reason, it is imperative that molecular sequence-based approaches be validated and used in prospective trials to achieve a better understanding of the bacterial characteristics associated with bacteremia of oral origin.
2. The prevention of bacteremia of oral origin has mostly focused on the use of antibiotic prophylaxis prior to dental extractions. However, when comparing antibiotics, there are important differences with respect to the type and dose of antibiotic used, and time of administration. Penicillins have been the most-studied antibiotics for bacteremia prophylaxis both by oral and parenteral routes. The doses and time of administration vary from 1–3 g and 1–2 hours, respectively for the oral route, which has been the best-studied route of administration. In the majority of studies, penicillins were effective at reducing bacteremia after a dental manipulation with respect to the placebo or control. However, clindamycin, azithromycin and cephalosporin have been suggested as alternatives in allergic patients, although fewer studies have been performed on their prophylactic efficacy.
3. Some Expert Committees have recommended another complementary method for the prevention of bacteremia of oral origin, which is antiseptic prophylaxis. Numerous studies exist concerning its efficacy at preventing bacteremia secondary to dental procedures. However, comparisons reveal significant methodological differences relating to the dental treatment, the type of antiseptic used and its concentration, as well as the application technique of the antiseptic solution (mouthwash, toothbrush and/or irrigation). The mouthwashes, performed individually or in combination with irrigation, have been the best-studied application technique. Regarding the antiseptic protocol, chlorhexidine has been the best-tested antimicrobial agent, although povidone iodine and essential oils appear to be possible options. However, none of them has been demonstrated to be clearly effective at reducing bacteremia secondary to dental procedures.

Nowadays, the controversies concerning the efficacy of antibiotic prophylaxis and the risk/cost-benefit relationships of antibiotic prophylaxis might justify the convenience of more extensive research on the recommended chlorhexidine regimens and new antiseptic protocols, specifically analysing their effect on the magnitude and duration of bacteremia of oral origin.

4. In general terms, further evidence-based well-designed research on the efficacy of antimicrobials in the prevention of oral bacteraemic episodes is needed. This is in order to reach a major consensus in the scientific community on the antimicrobial prophylaxis of potential complications, derived from a bacteremia of oral origin.

References

[1] Socransky SS, Manganiello SD. The oral microbiota of man from birth to senility. *Journal of Periodontology* 1971; 42:485-96.

[2] Aas JA, Paster BJ, Stokes LN, Olsen I, Dewhirst FE. Defining the normal bacterial flora of the oral cavity. *Journal of Clinical Microbiology* 2005; 43:5721-32.

[3] Kinane DF, Riggio MP, Walker KF, MacKenzie D, Shearer B. Bacteremia following periodontal procedures. *Journal of Clinical Periodontology* 2005; 32:708-13.

[4] Lockhart PB, Brennan MT, Sasser HC, Fox PC, Paster BJ, Bahrani-Mougeot FK. Bacteremia associated with toothbrushing and dental extraction. *Circulation* 2008; 117:3118-25.

[5] Savarrio L, Mackenzie D, Riggio M, Saunders WP, Bagg J. Detection of bacteremias during non-surgical root canal treatment. *Journal of Dentistry* 2005; 33:293-303.

[6] Sonbol H, Spratt D, Roberts GJ, Lucas VS. Prevalence, intensity and identity of bacteremia following conservative dental procedures in children. *Oral Microbiology and Immunology* 2009; 24:177-82.

[7] Benitez-Paez A, Álvarez M, Belda-Ferre P, Rubido S, Mira A, Tomás I. Detection of transient bacteremia following dental extractions by 16S rDNA pyrosequencing: a pilot study. *PLoS One* 2013; 8:e57782.

[8] Costerton JW, Stewart PS, Greenberg EP. Bacterial biofilms: a common cause of persistent infections. *Science* 1999; 284:1318-22.

[9] Slavkin HC. Biofilms, microbial ecology and Antoni van Leeuwenhoek. *Journal of the American Dental Association* 1997; 128:492-5.

[10] Parahitiyawa NB, Jin LJ, Leung WK, Yam WC, Samaranayake LP. Microbiology of odontogenic bacteremia: beyond endocarditis. *Clinical Microbiology Reviews* 2009; 22:46-64.

[11] Poveda-Roda R, Jiménez Y, Carbonell E, Gavalda C, Margaix-Muñoz MM, Sarrión-Pérez G. Bacteremia originating in the oral cavity. A review. *Medicina Oral Patología Oral y Cirugía Bucal* 2008; 13:E355-62.

[12] Everett ED, Hirschmann JV. Transient bacteremia and endocarditis prophylaxis. *A review. Medicine* (Baltimore) 1977; 56:61-77.

[13] Bristish Cardiac Society Clinical Practice Committee & Royal College of Physicians. Dental aspects of endocarditis prophylaxis: *new recommendations from a Working 30 Group of the Bristish Cardiac Society Clinical Practice Committee and Royal College of Physicians Clinical Effectiveness and Evaluation.* 2004: from: http://www.bcs.com/library.

[14] Osler W. The Gulstonian Lectures, on Malignant Endocarditis. *British Medical Journal* 1885; 1:467-70.

[15] Okell CC, Elliott SD. Bacteremia and oral sepsis with special reference to the aetiology of subacute endocarditis. *Lancet* 1935; 2:869-72.

[16] Burket LW, Burn CG. Bacteremias following dental extraction. Demonstration of source of bacteria by means of a non-pathogen (Serratia marcescens). *Journal of Dental Research* 1937; 16:521-30.

[17] Bender IB, Pressman RS. Factors in dental bacteremia. *Journal of the American Dental Association* 1945; 32:836-53.

[18] Heimdahl A, Hall G, Hedberg M, Sandberg H, Soder PO, Tuner K, et al. Detection and quantitation by lysis-filtration of bacteremia after different oral surgical procedures. *Journal of Clinical Microbiology* 1990; 28: 2205-9.

[19] Tuna A, Delilbasi C, Arslan A, Gurol Y, Tazegun Tekkanat Z. Do antibacterial mouthrinses affect bacteremia in third molar surgery? A pilot study. *Australian Dental Journal* 2012; 57:435-9.

[20] Elliott RH, Dunbar JM. Streptococcal bacteremia in children following dental extractions. *Archives of Disease in Childhood* 1968; 43:451-4.

[21] Shanson DC, Cannon P, Wilks M. Amoxycillin compared with penicillin V for the prophylaxis of dental bacteremia. *Journal of Antimicrobial Therapy* 1978; 4:431-6.

[22] Cannell H, Kerawala C, Sefton AM, Maskell JP, Seymour A, Sun ZM, et al. Failure of two macrolide antibiotics to prevent post-extraction bacteremia. *British Dental Journal* 1991; 171:170-3.

[23] Rajasuo A, Nyfors S, Kanervo A, Jousimies-Somer H, Lindqvist C, Suuronen R. Bacteremia after plate removal and tooth extraction. *International Journal of Oral Maxillofacial Surgery* 2004; 33:356-60.

[24] Tomás I, Pereira F, Llucian R, Poveda R, Diz P, Bagán JV. Prevalence of bacteremia following third molar surgery. *Oral Diseases* 2008; 14: 89-94.

[25] Diz Dios P, Tomás Carmona I, Limeres Posse J, Medina Henríquez J, Fernández Feijoo J, Álvarez Fernández M. Comparative efficacies of amoxicillin, clindamycin, and moxifloxacin in prevention of bacteremia following dental extractions. *Antimicrobial Agents and Chemotherapy* 2006; 50:2996-3002.

[26] Bahrani-Mougeot FK, Paster BJ, Coleman S, Ashar J, Barbuto S, Lockhart PB. Diverse and novel oral bacterial species in blood following dental procedures. *Journal of Clinical Microbiology* 2008; 46:2129-32.

[27] Rahman N, Rogers S, Ryan D, Healy C, Flint S. Infective endocarditis prophylaxis and the current AHA, BSAC, NICE and Australian guidelines. *Journal of the Irish Dental Association* 2008; 54:264-70.

[28] Heimdahl A, Josefsson K, von Konow L, Nord CE. Detection of anaerobic bacteria in blood cultures by lysis filtration. *European Journal of Clinical Microbiology* 1985; 4:404-7.

[29] Roberts GJ, Holzel HS, Sury MR, Simmons NA, Gardner P, Longhurst P. Dental bacteremia in children. *Pediatric Cardiology* 1997; 18:24-7.

[30] Tomás I, Álvarez M, Limeres J, Tomás M, Medina J, Otero JL, et al. Effect of a chlorhexidine mouthwash on the risk of postextraction bacteremia. *Infection Control and Hospital Epidemiology* 2007; 28:577-82.

[31] Okabe K, Nakagawa K, Yamamoto E. Factors affecting the occurrence of bacteremia associated with tooth extraction. *International Journal of Oral Maxillofacial Surgery* 1995; 24:239-42.

[32] Robinson L, Kraus FW, Lazansky JP, Wheeler RE, Gordon S, Johnson V. Bacteremias of dental origin. II. A study of the factors influencing occurrence and detection. *Oral Surgery* 1950; 3:923-6.

[33] Dajani AS, Taubert KA, Wilson W, Bolger AF, Bayer A, Ferrieri P, et al. Prevention of bacterial endocarditis: recommendations by the American Heart Association. *Journal of the American Dental Association* 1997; 128:1142-51.

[34] Lucas V, Roberts GJ. Odontogenic bacteremia following tooth cleaning procedures in children. *Pediatric Dentistry* 2000; 22:96-100.

[35] Roberts GJ. Dentists are innocent! "Everyday" bacteremia is the real culprit: a review and assessment of the evidence that dental surgical procedures are a principal cause of bacterial endocarditis in children. *Pediatric Cardiology* 1999; 20:317-25.

[36] Danchin N, Duval X, Leport C. Prophylaxis of infective endocarditis: French recommendations 2002. *Heart* 2005; 91:715-8.

[37] Durack DT. Infective and non-infective endocarditis. In: Schlant R, Alexander RW, editors. *The Heart: Arteries and Veins*. 8th ed. New York: McGraw-Hill; 1994. p. 1681–709.

[38] Glenny AM, Oliver R, Roberts GJ, Hooper L, Worthington HV. Antibiotics for the prophylaxis of bacterial endocarditis in dentistry. *Cochrane Database of Systematic Reviews* 2013; 10:CD003813.

[39] Gendron R, Grenier D, Maheu-Robert L. The oral cavity as a reservoir of bacterial pathogens for focal infections. *Microbes and Infection* 2000; 2:897-906.

[40] Bennis A, Zahraoui M, Azzouzi L, Soulami S, Mehadji BA, Tahiri A, et al. [Bacterial endocarditis in Morocco]. *Annales de Cardiologie et d'Angéiologie* (Paris) 1995; 44:339-44.

[41] Shrihari TG. Potential correlation between periodontitis and coronary heart disease--an overview. *General Dentistry* 2012; 60:20-4.

[42] Olsen I. Update on bacteremia related to dental procedures. *Transfusion and Apheresis Science* 2008; 39:173-8.

[43] Tomás Carmona I, Diz Dios P, Limeres Posse J, González Quintela A, Martínez Vázquez C, Castro Iglesias A. An update on infective endocarditis of dental origin. *Journal of Dentistry* 2002; 30:37-40.

[44] Limeres J, Tomás I, Feijoo JF, Martínez C, Castro A, Diz P, et al. Abscesos cerebrales de origen oral. *Revista de Neurología* 2003; 37:201.

[45] American Heart Association. Prevention of Rheumatic Fever and Bacterial Endocarditis through Control of Streptococcal Infections. *Circulation* 1955; 11:317-20.

[46] Thornhill MH, Dayer MJ, Forde JM, Corey GR, Chu VH, Couper DJ, et al. Impact of the NICE guideline recommending cessation of antibiotic prophylaxis for prevention of infective endocarditis: before and after study. *British Medical Journal* 2011; 342:d2392.

[47] Wilson W, Taubert KA, Gewitz M, Lockhart PB, Baddour LM, Levison M, et al. Prevention of infective endocarditis: guidelines from the American Heart Association: a guideline from the American Heart

Association Rheumatic Fever, Endocarditis, and Kawasaki Disease Committee, Council on Cardiovascular Disease in the Young, and the Council on Clinical Cardiology, Council on Cardiovascular Surgery and Anesthesia, and the Quality of Care and Outcomes Research Interdisciplinary Working Group. *Circulation* 2007; 116:1736-54.

[48] Lockhart PB, Blizzard J, Maslow AL, Brennan MT, Sasser H, Carew J. Drug cost implications for antibiotic prophylaxis for dental procedures. Oral Surgery, Oral Medicine, *Oral Pathology and Oral Radiology* 2013; 115: 345-53.

[49] Bhayat A, Jarab F, Mansuri S, Ahmad MS, Mahrous MS. Assessment of knowledge of dental staff at a saudi arabian university regarding the prophylaxis for infective endocarditis. *The Open Dentistry Journal* 2013; 7:82-7.

[50] Gould FK, Elliott TS, Foweraker J, Fulford M, Perry JD, Roberts GJ, et al. Guidelines for the prevention of endocarditis: report of the Working Party of the British Society for Antimicrobial Chemotherapy. *Journal of Antimicrobial Therapy* 2006; 57:1035-42.

[51] Horstkotte D, Follath F, Gutschik E, Lengyel M, Oto A, Pavie A, et al. Guidelines on prevention, diagnosis and treatment of infective endocarditis executive summary; the task force on infective endocarditis of the European society of cardiology. *European Heart Journal* 2004; 25: 267-76.

[52] Simmons NA, Cawson RA, Clarke C. The antibiotic prophylaxis of infective endocarditis. Report of a working party of the British Society for Antimicrobial Chemotherapy. *Lancet* 1982; 2:1323-6.

[53] The Centre for Clinical Practice at NICE. Prophylaxis against Infective Endocarditis: *Antimicrobial Prophylaxis Against Infective Endocarditis in Adults and Children Undergoing Interventional Procedures.* London 2008.

[54] Delahaye F, De Gevigney G. Should we give antibiotic prophylaxis against infective endocarditis in all cardiac patients, whatever the type of dental treatment? *Heart* 2001; 85:9-10.

[55] Glauser MP, Bernard JP, Moreillon P, Francioli P. Successful single-dose amoxicillin prophylaxis against experimental streptococcal endocarditis: evidence for two mechanisms of protection. *Journal of Infectious Diseases* 1983; 147:568-75.

[56] Berney P, Francioli P. Successful prophylaxis of experimental streptococcal endocarditis with single-dose amoxicillin administered

after bacterial challenge. *Journal of Infectious Diseases* 1990; 161: 281-5.

[57] Dall L, Keilhofner M, Herndon B, Barnes W, Lane J. Clindamycin effect on glycocalyx production in experimental viridans streptococcal endocarditis. *Journal of Infectious Diseases* 1990; 161:1221-4.

[58] Little J. The American Heart Association's guidelines for the prevention of bacterial endocarditis: a critical review. *General Dentistry* 1998; 46: 508-15.

[59] Mizen L, Woodnutt G. A critique of animal pharmacokinetics. *Journal of Antimicrobial Therapy* 1988; 21:273-8.

[60] Vogelman B, Gudmundsson S, Leggett J, Turnidge J, Ebert S, Craig WA. Correlation of antimicrobial pharmacokinetic parameters with therapeutic efficacy in an animal model. *Journal of Infectious Diseases* 1988; 158:831-47.

[61] Durack DT. Prevention of infective endocarditis. *New England Journal of Medicine* 1995; 332:38-44.

[62] Oliver R, Roberts GJ, Hooper L, Worthington HV. Antibiotics for the prophylaxis of bacterial endocarditis in dentistry. *Cochrane Database of Systematic Reviews* 2008:CD003813.

[63] Segreti J. Is antibiotic prophylaxis necessary for preventing prosthetic device infection? *Infectious Disease Clinics of North America* 1999; 13:871-7, vii.

[64] Van der Meer JT, Van Wijk W, Thompson J, Vandenbroucke JP, Valkenburg HA, Michel MF. Efficacy of antibiotic prophylaxis for prevention of native-valve endocarditis. *Lancet* 1992; 339:135-9.

[65] Strom BL, Abrutyn E, Berlin JA, Kinman JL, Feldman RS, Stolley PD, et al. Dental and cardiac risk factors for infective endocarditis. A population-based, case-control study. *Annals of Internal Medicine* 1998; 129:761-9.

[66] Shanson DC, Akash S, Harris M, Tadayon M. Erythromycin stearate, 1.5 g, for the oral prophylaxis of streptococcal bacteremia in patients undergoing dental extraction: efficacy and tolerance. *Journal of Antimicrobial Therapy* 1985; 15:83-90.

[67] Roberts GJ, Radford P, Holt R. Prophylaxis of dental bacteremia with oral amoxycillin in children. *British Dental Journal* 1987; 162:179-82.

[68] Göker K, Güvener O. Antibacterial effects of ofloxacin, clindamycin and sultamicillin on surgical removal of impacted third molars. *Journal of Marmara University Dental Faculty* 1992; 1:237-49.

[69] Hall G, Hedstrom SA, Heimdahl A, Nord CE. Prophylactic administration of penicillins for endocarditis does not reduce the incidence of postextraction bacteremia. *Clinical Infectious Disease* 1993; 17:188-94.

[70] Josefsson K, Heimdahl A, von Konow L, Nord CE. Effect of phenoxymethylpenicillin and erythromycin prophylaxis on anaerobic bacteremia after oral surgery. *Journal of Antimicrobial Therapy* 1985; 16:243-51.

[71] Sefton AM, Maskell JP, Kerawala C, Cannell H, Seymour A, Sun ZM, et al. Comparative efficacy and tolerance of erythromycin and josamycin in the prevention of bacteremia following dental extraction. *Journal of Antimicrobial Therapy* 1990; 25:975-84.

[72] Aitken C, Cannell H, Sefton AM, Kerawala C, Seymour A, Murphy M, et al. Comparative efficacy of oral doses of clindamycin and erythromycin in the prevention of bacteremia. *British Dental Journal* 1995; 178:418-22.

[73] Hall G, Nord CE, Heimdahl A. Elimination of bacteremia after dental extraction: comparison of erythromycin and clindamycin for prophylaxis of infective endocarditis. *Journal of Antimicrobial Therapy* 1996; 37:783-95.

[74] Vergis EN, Demas PN, Vaccarello SJ, Yu VL. Topical antibiotic prophylaxis for bacteremia after dental extractions. *Oral Surgery, Oral Medicine, Oral Pathology, Oral Radiology and Endodontology* 2001; 91:162-5.

[75] Lockhart PB, Brennan MT, Kent ML, Norton HJ, Weinrib DA. Impact of amoxicillin prophylaxis on the incidence, nature, and duration of bacteremia in children after intubation and dental procedures. *Circulation* 2004; 109:2878-84.

[76] Hess J, Holloway Y, Dankert J. Incidence of postextraction bacteremia under penicillin cover in children with cardiac disease. *Pediatrics* 1983; 71:554-8.

[77] Kaneko A, Sasaki J, Yamazaki J, Kobayashi I. Intravenous administration of vancomycin is ineffective against bacteremia following tooth extraction. *The Tokai Journal of Experimental and Clinical Medicine* 1995; 20:65-6.

[78] Roberts G, Holzel H. Intravenous antibiotic regimens and prophylaxis of odontogenic bacteremia. *British Dental Journal* 2002; 193:525-7; discussion 18.

[79] Baltch AL, Schaffer C, Hammer MC, SutphenNT, Smith RP, Conroy J, et al. Bacteremia following dental cleaning in patients with and without penicillin prophylaxis. *American Heart Journal* 1982; 104:1335-9.

[80] Baltch AL, Pressman HL, Hammer MC, Sutphen NC, Smith RP, Shayegani M. Bacteremia following dental extractions in patients with and without penicillin prophylaxis. *American Journal of the Medical Sciences* 1982; 283: 129-40.

[81] Morozumi T, Kubota T, Abe D, Shimizu T, Komatsu Y, Yoshie H. Effects of irrigation with an antiseptic and oral administration of azithromycin on bacteremia caused by scaling and root planing. *Journal of Periodontology* 2010; 81:1555-63.

[82] Maharaj B, Coovadia Y, Vayej AC. A comparative study of amoxicillin, clindamycin and chlorhexidine in the prevention of post-extraction bacteremia. *Cardiovascular Journal of Africa* 2012; 23:491-4.

[83] Duvall NB, Fisher TD, Hensley D, Hancock RH, VandewalleKS. The comparative efficacy of 0.12% chlorhexidine and amoxicillin to reduce the incidence and magnitude of bacteremia during third molar extractions: a prospective, blind, randomized clinical trial. *Oral Surgery, Oral Medicine, Oral Pathology and Oral Radiology* 2013; 115:752-63.

[84] Bartlett RC, Howell RM. Topical vancomycin as a deterrent to bacteremias following dental procedures. *Oral Surgery, Oral Medicine, Oral Pathology and Oral Radiology* 1973; 35:780-8.

[85] Head TW, Bentley KC, Millar EP, deVries JA. A comparative study of the effectiveness of metronidazole and penicillin V in eliminating anaerobes from postextraction bacteremias. *Oral Surgery, Oral Medicine, Oral Pathology and Oral Radiology* 1984; 58:152-5.

[86] Shanson DC, Shehata A, Tadayon M, Harris M. Comparison of intravenous teicoplanin with intramuscular amoxycillin for the prophylaxis of streptococcal bacteremia in dental patients. *Journal of Antimicrobial Therapy* 1987; 20:85-93.

[87] Hall G, Heimdahl A, Nord CE. Effects of prophylactic administration of cefaclor on transient bacteremia after dental extraction. *European Journal of Clinical Microbiology Infectious Disease* 1996; 15: 646-9.

[88] Wahlmann U, Al-Nawas B, Jutte M, Wagner W. Clinical and microbiological efficacy of single dose cefuroxime prophylaxis for dental surgical procedures. *International Journal of Antimicrobial Agents* 1999; 12:253-6.

[89] Brennan MT, Kent ML, Fox PC, Norton HJ, Lockhart PB. The impact of oral disease and nonsurgical treatment on bacteremia in children. *Journal of the American Dental Association* 2007; 138:80-5.

[90] Bender IB, Pressman RS. Antibiotic treatment of the gingival sulcus in prevention of postextraction bacteremia. *Journal of Oral Surgery* (Chic) 1956; 14:20-8.

[91] DrangsholtMT. A new causal model of dental diseases associated with endocarditis. *Annals of Periodontology* 1998; 3:184-96.

[92] Jokinen MA. Prevention of postextraction bacteremia by local prophylaxis. *International Journal of Oral Surgery* 1978; 7:450-2.

[93] Macfarlane TW, Ferguson MM, Mulgrew CJ. Post-extraction bacteremia: role of antiseptics and antibiotics. *British Dental Journal* 1984; 156:179-81.

[94] Bolukbasi N, Ozdemir T, Oksuz L, Gurler N. Bacteremia following dental implant surgery: preliminary results. *Medicina Oral, Patologia Oral y Cirugia Bucal* 2012; 17:69-75.

[95] Durack DT. Antibiotics for prevention of endocarditis during dentistry: time to scale back? *Annals of Internal Medicine* 1998; 129:829-31.

[96] Lowy FD, Neuhaus EG, Chang DS, Steigbigel NH. Penicillin therapy of experimental endocarditis induced by tolerant Streptococcus sanguis and nontolerant Streptococcus mitis. *Antimicrobial Agents and Chemotherapy* 1983; 23:67-73.

[97] Bender IB, Naidorf IJ, Garvey GJ. Bacterial endocarditis: a consideration for physician and dentist. *Journal of the American Dental Association* 1984; 109:415-20.

[98] Longman LP, Martin MV, Smalley JW. One and two doses of cephradine in the prophylaxis of experimental streptococcal endocarditis. *Journal of Antimicrobial Therapy* 1987; 20:557-62.

[99] García E, Azanza JR, Pérez JH. Antibióticos en Odontoestomatología y Cirugía Maxilofacial. Estructura química y principios básicos farmacocinéticos. In: Liébana Ureña J, Bagán Sebastián JV, editors. *Terapéutica antimicrobiana en Odontoestomatología*. Madrid: IM&C; 1996. p. 59-99.

[100] Moreillon P, Francioli P, Overholser D, Meylan P, Glauser MP. Mechanisms of successful amoxicillin prophylaxis of experimental endocarditis due to Streptococcus intermedius. *Journal of Infectious Diseases* 1986; 154:801-7.

[101] Fluckiger U, Moreillon P, Blaser J, Bickle M, Glauser MP, Francioli P. Simulation of amoxicillin pharmacokinetics in humans for the

prevention of streptococcal endocarditis in rats. *Antimicrobial Agents and Chemotherapy* 1994; 38:2846-9.

[102] Habib G, Hoen B, Tornos P, Thuny F, Prendergast B, Vilacosta I, et al. Guidelines on the prevention, diagnosis, and treatment of infective endocarditis (new version 2009): the Task Force on the Prevention, Diagnosis, and Treatment of Infective Endocarditis of the European Society of Cardiology (ESC). Endorsed by the European Society of Clinical Microbiology and Infectious Diseases (ESCMID) and the International Society of Chemotherapy (ISC) for Infection and Cancer. *European Heart Journal* 2009; 30:2369-413.

[103] Addy M, Jenkins S, Newcombe R. The effect of some chlorhexidine-containing mouthrinses on salivary bacterial counts. *Journal of Clinical Periodontology* 1991; 18:90-3.

[104] Jenkins S, Addy M, Wade W, Newcombe RG. The magnitude and duration of the effects of some mouthrinse products on salivary bacterial counts. *Journal of Clinical Periodontology* 1994; 21: 397-401.

[105] Netuschil L, Reich E, Brecx M. Direct measurement of the bactericidal effect of chlorhexidine on human dental plaque. *Journal of Clinical Periodontology* 1989; 16:484-8.

[106] Konig J, Storcks V, Kocher T, Bossmann K, Plagmann HC. Anti-plaque effect of tempered 0.2% chlorhexidine rinse: an *in vivo* study. *Journal of Clinical Periodontology* 2002; 29:207-10.

[107] Barros VMR, Ito IY, Azevedo RVP, Morello D, Rosateli PAl. Estudo comparativo da eficiência de três métodos de anti-sepsia intrabucal na reduçao do número de estreptococos do sulco gengiva. *Revista de Odontologia da Universidade de Sao Paulo* 1998; 12:201-6.

[108] Lockhart PB. An analysis of bacteremias during dental extractions. A double-blind, placebo-controlled study of chlorhexidine. *Archives of Internal Medicine* 1996; 156:513-20.

[109] Brown AR, Papasian CJ, Shultz P, Theisen FC, Shultz RE. Bacteremia and intraoral suture removal: can an antimicrobial rinse help? *Journal of the American Dental Association* 1998; 129:1455-61.

[110] Rise E, Smith JF, Bell J. Reduction of bacteremia after oral manipulations. *Archives Of Otolaryngology* (Chicago, III: 1960) 1969; 90:198-201.

[111] Keosian J, Rafel S, Weinman I. The effect of aqueous diatomic iodine mouth washes on the incidence of postextraction bacteremia. *Oral Surgery, Oral Medicine and Oral Pathology* 1956; 9:1337-41.

[112] Jones JC, Cutcher JL, Goldberg. Control of bacteremia associated with extraction of teeth. *Oral Surgery, Oral Medicine and Oral Pathology* 1970; 30:454-9.

[113] Scopp IW, Orvieto LD. Gingival degerming by povidone-iodine irrigation: bacteremia reduction in extraction procedures. *Journal of the American Dental Association* 1971; 83:1294-6.

[114] Huffman GG, Wood WH, Hausler WJ, Jensen J. The effects of preoperative rinsing with cetylpyridinium chloride on bacteremia associated with the surgical removal of impacted third molars. *Oral Surgery, Oral Medicine and Oral Pathology* 1974; 38:359-66.

[115] Sweet JB, Gill VJ, Chusid MJ, Elin RJ. Nitroblue tetrazolium and Limulus assays for bacteremia after dental extraction: effect of topical antiseptics. *Journal of the American Dental Association* 1978; 96:276-81.

[116] Witzenberger T, O'Leary TJ, Gillette WB. Effect of a local germicide on the occurrence of bacteremia during subgingival scaling. *Journal of Periodontology* 1982; 53:172-9.

[117] Lofthus JE, Waki MY, Jolkovsky DL, Otomo-Corgel J, Newman MG, Flemmig T, et al. Bacteremia following subgingival irrigation and scaling and root planing. *Journal of Periodontology* 1991; 62:602-7.

[118] Allison C, Simor AE, Mock D, Tenenbaum HC. Prosol-chlorhexidine irrigation reduces the incidence of bacteremia during ultrasonic scaling with the Cavi-Med: a pilot investigation. *Journal of the Canadian Dental Association* 1993; 59:673, 6-82.

[119] Rahn R, Schneider S, Diehl O, Schafer V, Shah PM. Preventing post-treatment bacteremia: comparing topical povidone-iodine and chlorhexidine. *Journal of the American Dental Association* 1995; 126:1145-9.

[120] Fine DH, Korik I, Furgang D, Myers R, Olshan A, Barnett ML, et al. Assessing pre-procedural subgingival irrigation and rinsing with an antiseptic mouthrinse to reduce bacteremia. *Journal of the American Dental Association* 1996; 127:641-2, 5-6.

[121] Erverdi N, Acar A, Isguden B, Kadir T. Investigation of bacteremia after orthodontic banding and debanding following chlorhexidine mouth wash application. *The Angle Orthodontist* 2001; 71:190-4.

[122] Cherry M, Daly CG, Mitchell D, Highfield J. Effect of rinsing with povidone-iodine on bacteremia due to scaling: a randomized-controlled trial. *Journal of Clinical Periodontology* 2007; 34:148-55.

[123] Fine DH, Furgang D, McKiernan M, Tereski-Bischio D, Ricci-Nittel D, Zhang P, et al. An investigation of the effect of an essential oil mouthrinse on induced bacteremia: a pilot study. *Journal of Clinical Periodontology* 2010; 37:840-7.

[124] Piñeiro A, Tomás I, Blanco J, Alvarez M, Seoane J, Diz P. Bacteremia following dental implants' placement. *Clinical Oral Implants Research* 2010; 21:913-8.

[125] Madsen KL. Effect of chlorhexidine mouthrinse and periodontal treatment upon bacteremia produced by oral hygiene procedures. *Scandinavian Journal of Dental Research* 1974; 82:1-7.

[126] Cortelli JR, Cogo K, Aquino DR, Cortelli SC, Ricci-Nittel D, Zhang P, et al. Validation of the anti-bacteremic efficacy of an essential oil rinse in a Brazilian population: a cross-over study. *Brazilian Oral Research* 2012; 26:478-84.

[127] Waki MY, Jolkovsky DL, Otomo-Corgel J, Lofthus JE, Nachnani S, Newman MG, et al. Effects of subgingival irrigation on bacteremia following scaling and root planing. *Journal of Periodontology* 1990; 61:405-11.

[128] Erverdi N, Kadir T, Ozkan H, Acar A. Investigation of bacteremia after orthodontic banding. *American Journal of Orthodontics and Dentofacial Orthopedics: Official Publication of the American Association of Orthodontists, Its Constituent Societies, and the American Board of Orthodontics* 1999; 116:687-90.

[129] Erverdi N, Biren S, Kadir T, Acar A. Investigation of bacteremia following orthodontic debanding. *The Angle Orthodontist* 2000; 70:11-4; discussion 5.

[130] Jones CG. Chlorhexidine: is it still the gold standard? *Periodontology 2000* 1997; 15:55-62.

[131] Shen Y, Stojicic S, Haapasalo M. Antimicrobial efficacy of chlorhexidine against bacteria in biofilms at different stages of development. *Journal of Endodontics* 2011; 37:657-61.

[132] Eick S, Goltz S, Nietzsche S, Jentsch H, Pfister W. Efficacy of chlorhexidine digluconate-containing formulations and other mouthrinses against periodontopathogenic microorganisms. *Quintessence International* 2011; 42:687-700.

In: Bacteremia
Editor: Jodie P. Williams

ISBN: 978-1-63117-290-8

Chapter IV

Bacterial Sepsis and Perioperative Nutritional Support Therapy in Living Donor Liver Transplantation

Noboru Harada*[*]*, M.D., Ken Shirabe, M.D., Yuji Soejima, M.D.,Tomoharu Yoshizumi, M.D., Toru Ikegami, M.D., Hideaki Uchiyama, M.D., Yo-ichi Yamashita, M.D., Mizuki Ninomiya, M.D., Hirofumi Kawanaka, M.D., Tomohiko Akahoshi, M.D., and Yoshihiko Maehara, M.D.

Department of Surgery and Science,
Graduate School of Medical Sciences, Kyushu University

[*] Correspondence and reprint requests to: Noboru Harada, MD. PhD. Department of Surgery and Science, Graduate School of Medical Sciences, Kyushu University, 3-1-1, Maidashi, Higashi-ku, Fukuoka, 812-8582, Japan. Phone: 81-92-642-5466, Fax: 81-92-642-5482. E-mail: noharada14@yahoo.co.jp.

Abstract

Bacterial sepsis is a frequent occurrence during the first 1–2 months after liver transplantation under immunosuppressive therapy. Despite recent advances in perioperative management and surgical techniques, postoperative mortality and morbidity rates are still associated with infectious complications, such as bacterial sepsis, after liver transplantation. Furthermore, bacterial sepsis is the most frequent cause of in-hospital death after living donor liver transplantation (LDLT).

In this chapter, the etiology, outcomes, and risk factors of bacterial sepsis after LDLT are discussed. In addition, we focus on the effect of perioperative nutritional support in LDLT for preventing bacterial sepsis after LDLT. LDLT involves a smaller graft size and scheduled non-emergent surgery compared with deceased donor liver transplantation. A smaller graft size is the main disadvantage of adult-to-adult LDLT because it results in increased portal venous pressure, impaired bowel motility, bacterial translocation, ascites production, and hyperbilirubinemia.

In the last 2 decades, nutritional support has been recognized as a vital component for the management of critically ill patients, by delivering preoperative essential substrates and nutrition using enteral feeding, to aid patient recovery. In particular, preoperative branched-chain amino acid supplementation might reduce the incidence of postoperative bacterial sepsis after LDLT. Additionally, early enteral nutrition is associated with a significantly reduced risk of developing bacterial sepsis after LDLT.

Therefore, poor nutritional status of pre-transplants can be improved by using nutritional support, and the high infectious status of post-transplants under immunosuppressive therapy can be improved with initiation of early postoperative enteral nutrition. Improved nutrition supports a functional immune system, and reduces septic morbidity and mortality in patients with liver transplantation.

Abbreviations

LDLT	living donor liver transplantation
BCAA	branched-chain amino acid
SGOT	serum glutamic oxalacetic transaminase
SGPT	serum glutamic pyruvic transaminase
I.U.	international unit
TMP/SMX	trimethoprim-sulfamethoxazole

MINO	minocycline hydrochloride
PMX	polymyxin B
CHDF	continuous hemodiafiltration
ESLD	end-stage liver disease
ESPEN	European Society for Clinical Nutrition and Metabolism
SGA	subjective global assessment
DEXA	dual energy X-ray absorptiometry
BMC	body cell mass
BIA	bioelectrical impedance analysis
ASPEN	American Society for Parenteral and Enteral Nutrition
ICU	intensive care unit
MUST	Malnutrition Universal Screening Tool
BMI	body mass index

Etiology, Outcomes and Risk Factors of Bacterial Sepsis After Liver Transplantation

Bacterial sepsis occurs after liver transplantation because the host immune system against bacterial species is defenseless under various postoperative complications owing to strong immunosuppressive therapy. Starzl et al. first reported three patients with liver sepsis after homotransplantations of the human liver in 1968 [1]. In their report, all three transplants developed life-threatening infections in the homografts coincident with Gram-negative septicemia. In patient 1, 23 days after the operation, she developed hypotension and a fever of a 41°C. Blood cultures at this time and 12 hours later contained *Escherichia coli*. A repeated liver scan showed a large, filling defect in the right lobe. This child was treated for the next week with intravenous kanamycin, polymyxin, and ampicillin, but in this interval, *Aerobacter-Klebsiella* was found in two other blood cultures. Consequently, the cause of sepsis was necrosis in the right lobe of the liver and she improved after surgical treatment for this area. Patient 2, who received a homograft with a double arterial supply, immediately developed an infarct of the posterior segment of the right liver lobe. *Bacteroides fragilis*, which was sensitive only to tetracycline, was cultured from her blood. Eight days after transplantation, the original incision was reopened and a posterior segmentectomy was carried out. Two weeks later, it was re-drained laterally through the 10th intercostal space because of evidence of residual fluid collection and there were several more blood cultures positive for Bacteroides. Subsequent wound management was similar to that in Patient 1. In the third case, a culture of the recipient duodenum at the time of homotransplantation showed *Aerobacter-Klebsiella*. Antibiotic therapy was provided. However, on the 25th day post-operation, the patient developed Gram-negative septicemia with *Aerobacter-Klebsiella*, hypoglycemia, and respiratory arrest. After resuscitation, a liver scan showed a central defect in the right lobe, and within 2 days, it had spread to involve almost 25% of the liver. An emergency debridement procedure similar to that in Patient 1 was carried out laterally through the 10th intercostal space. All subsequent blood cultures were negative.

In each of these cases, there was marked improvement in the patient's condition after debridement procedures. These procedures were all carried out under heavy antibiotic coverage. Starzl et al. reported earlier [2, 3] that seven previous clinical attempts at orthotopic liver homotransplantations in their institution all resulted in early death of the recipients. Several changes in management probably contributed to survival in the three cases discussed above. A vital factor was the quality of the organs that were used. Every effort was made to maintain some circulation until these livers were cooled. In addition, the preservation system, which was used after the organs had been extirpated, is extremely effective. They succeeded in liver transplantation by these refinements, but bacterial sepsis was the most lethal complication under immunosuppressive therapy in these early days.

Harada et al. reported [4] a case of bacterial sepsis, *Stenotrophomonas maltophilia*, after living donor liver transplantation (LDLT). *Stenotrophomonas maltophilia* (previously named *Xanthomonas maltophilia*) is an aerobic, non-fermentive, Gram-negative bacillus that is widespread in the environment. This organism is considered to have a limited pathogenic potential, which is rarely capable of causing diseases in humans, other than in those who are in an immunocompromised state. *Stenotrophomonas maltophilia* shows clinical signs of severe sepsis and is resistant to almost all antibiotics. However, Harada et al. [4] successfully treated the patient with the antibiotics trimethoprim-sulfamethoxazole and minocycline hydrochloride, and performed endotoxin-absorbing therapy using polymyxin B to remove the endotoxin from the Gram-negative bacillus, as well as continuous hemodiafiltration to remove inflammatory cytokines. These refinements made it possible to treat the bacterial sepsis after liver transplantation.

Ikegami et al. reported [5] that 46 patients (13.3%) in 346 adult-to-adult LDLT experienced bacterial sepsis in our institution, with primary and secondary origins in 23.9% and 76.1% of patients, respectively. Gram-negative bacteria accounted for 71.7% of the bacteria isolated. The 2-year cumulative graft survival rate in patients with bacterial sepsis was 45.7%. Intraoperative massive blood loss >10 L (p<0.001) and no enteral feeding started within 48 hours after transplantation (p=0.005) were significant risk factors for bacterial sepsis.

Iida et al. [6] evaluated the risk factors for bacteremia after LDLT. One hundred and seventeen episodes of bacteremia occurred in 62 of 181 recipients (34.3%) within 12 days (median) after transplantation (range: 1–71 days). The most frequently isolated pathogens were *Pseudomonas aeruginosa* (26 episodes), methicillin-resistant coagulase-negative staphylococci (22 episodes), and *Enterococcus* sp. (11 episodes). The overall survival rate at 1 year for patients with bacteremia (n=62) was significantly lower than that for patients without bacteremia (n=119; 69.6% versus 92.3%, p<0.0001). Child-Pugh class C (p=0.0002), preoperative massive pleural effusion or ascites requiring drainage (p=0.0384), postoperative cytomegalovirus infection (p=0.0014), ABO incompatibility (p=0.0188), and older donor age (p=0.015) were independent risk factors for postoperative bacteremia.

Kim et al. reported [7] that among 144 consecutive LDLT recipients, 24% (34/144) developed bacteremia, 32% (46/144) developed non-bacteremic infections, and 44% (64/144) did not develop any infectious complications. Forty episodes of bacteremia occurred in 34 recipients. The major sources of bacteremia were intravascular catheters (30%; 12/40), the biliary tract (30%; 12/40), and the abdomen (22.5%; 9/40). Gram-positive cocci were more common (57.5%; 23/40) than Gram-negative rods (32.5%; 13/40) and fungi (10%; 4/40).

The risk factors for bacteremia were an age older than 55 years (odds ratio, 6.1; p=0.003), catheterization for more than 22 days (odds ratio, 4.0; p=0.009), UNOS class IIA (odds ratio, 6.6; p=0.039), and post-transplant hemodialysis (odds ratio, 23.1; p=0.001). One-year survival rates of the bacteremia, non-bacteremic infection, and no infection groups were 73.2%, 91.3%, and 93.5%, respectively. Therisk factors of bacterial sepsis after LDLT are shown in Table 1 [8, 9].

In this chapter, we focus on bacterial sepsis in LDLT. LDLT involves a smaller graft size and scheduled non-emergent surgery compared with deceased donor liver transplantation. Experimental and clinical evidence suggests that elevated portal pressure and portal over-perfusion form the central pathogenesis of the sequelae of small-for-size grafts [10-13].

A persistent elevation in portal pressure and resultant hyperperfusion of the graft are attributable to hyperdynamic splanchnic circulation and limited accommodation of the graft. This situation causes portal venular and sinusoidal endothelial injury and the release of deleterious mediators, which ultimately lead to serious graft injury [11].

Table 1. Risk factors of bacterial sepsis after living donor liver transplantation

Authors	Risk Factors
Ikegami T[5](2012)	intraoperative blood loss>10L, no posttransplant early enteral feeding
Rhee KW[8] (2012)	Age ≦1 year, bile duct complication (for pediatric transplants)
Iida T[6] (2010)	Child Pugh class C, preoperative massive pleural effusion or ascites requiring drainage, CMV infection, ABO incompatibility, older donor age
Kim SI[7] (2009)	older recipient age >55 years, catheterization for more than 22 days, UNOS class IIA, posttransplant hemodialysis
Hashimoto M[9](2008)	Diabetes mellitus, serum albumin level less than 2.4 g/dL

Therefore, a smaller graft size is the main disadvantage of adult-to-adult LDLT because it results in increased portal venous pressure. This leads to impaired bowel motility, bacterial translocation, ascites production, and hyperbilirubinemia, resulting in bacterial sepsis [5, 14].

Finally, bacterial sepsis after LDLT appears to be one of the most lethal complications and affects the prognosis of transplant recipients. To prevent postoperative bacterial sepsis from developing, there are many refinements of surgical and pre-and post-operative management.

Preoperative Nutritional Evaluation

There are many parameters, such as body weight, anthropometric measurements, creatinine-height index, nitrogen balance studies, 3-methylhistidine excretion, visceral protein levels, immune function tests, and bioelectrical impedance, that affect the interpretation of objective nutritional assessment tests in patients with liver cirrhosis. Sanchez et al. insisted [15] that a thorough clinical assessment must be performed, because many factors contribute to malnutrition in individuals with end-stage liver disease (ESLD), to determine the presence of malnutrition in patients with ESLD. In addition to a full medical history and physical examination, a complete dietary history is essential, preferably with the guidance of an experienced dietitian. Relevant details to medical records are the degree of anorexia, early satiety, weight changes, taste abnormalities, and the presence of chronic diarrhea. A physical exam may show subtle changes in oral mucosa, skin, and hair, which may indicate a deficiency in nutrients.

The European Society for Clinical Nutrition and Metabolism guideline recommended in 2006 [16] that undernutrition adversely affects the prognosis in transplant patients with liver cirrhosis. This guideline also stated that simple bedside methods, such as subjective global assessment or anthropometry, are considered adequate for identifying patients at risk. Accurate quantitative measurement of nutritional status is difficult in the presence of fluid overload or impaired hepatic protein synthesis (e.g., albumin). This necessitates sophisticated methods, such as total body potassium count, dual energy X-ray absorptiometry, *in vivo* neutron activation analysis, and isotope dilution. To quantitate undernutrition, determination of phase angle α or body cell mass using bioelectrical impedance analysis is recommended, despite some limitations in patients with ascites.

According to the American Society for Parenteral and Enteral Nutrition guideline in 2009 [17], the clinical consequences of liver failure render traditional nutrition assessment tools inaccurate and unreliable. Malnutrition is highly prevalent among patients withchronic liver disease and nearly universal among patients awaitingliver transplantation. The primary etiology of malnutrition is poor oralintake stemming from multiple factors. Malnutrition in patients with cirrhosis leads to increased morbidity and mortality rates. Furthermore, patients who are severely malnourished before transplant surgery havea higher rate of complications and a decreased overall survivalrate after liver transplantation.

Energy needs in criticallyill patients with liver disease are highly variable, are difficultto predict by simple equations in liver disease, and consequently, are best determined by indirect calorimetry in intensive care unit patientswith liver disease [16].

Another method for evaluating nutritional status is the Malnutrition Universal Screening Tool (MUST) (16), which provides a score that is based on the body mass index (<18.5, 18.5–20, or >20 kg/m^2), unplanned weight loss in a previous illness, or no nutritional intake for more than 5 days. The score categories are low risk (0), medium risk (1), and high risk (≥2).

Preoperative Nutritional Support, Including Branched-Chain Amino Acid Supplementation for Liver Transplantation

The nutritional status of patients with ESLD waiting for a liver transplant may deteriorate. The benefits of providing nutritional support to a preoperative recipient include enhanced immunological defense, improved wound healing, and replacement of energy stores. Sanchez et al. advocated [15] that the main goals of pre-transplant nutritional therapy are to prevent further nutrient and muscle depletion, and to correct any vitamin and mineral deficiencies present. They also argued that protein restriction should not be routinely performed in all patients with ESLD. Standard amino acid formulas are usually well tolerated, and branched amino acids should be considered only in patients with refractory encephalopathy. Protein intake should be at least 1g/kg/day initially, and then 24-hour urinary urea nitrogen can be measured to assess catabolic rate in patients with normal renal function. Progressive increments in protein supplementation should be implemented up to 1.8–2.0 g/kg/day as tolerated.

With regard to branched-chain amino acid (BCAA), Tietge et al. [18] investigated hepatic amino acid metabolism in patients with liver cirrhosis and over the long term after liver transplantation. They found that BCAA levels were lower in patients with liver cirrhosis. BCAA levels improved after orthotopic liver transplantation, although they were not normalized [18]. Other studies have shown that beneficial effects of BCAA supplementation prolong the time to liver transplantation by preserving hepatic functional reserve in patients with decompensated liver cirrhosis [19-23]. They also showed that oral BCAA supplementation restored serum bilirubin and albumin levels in a prospective, randomized trial [20, 21]. Furthermore, recent studies have shown that BCAAs restore the immune response in patients with decompensated liver cirrhosis [22, 23]. Because of these findings, BCAA supplementation for decompensated liver cirrhosis is becoming increasingly prevalent in Japan.

Shirabe et al. investigated the effects of preoperative oral supplementation with BCAAs on postoperative bacteremia after LDLT for chronic liver failure in our institution. Two hundred and thirty-six patients who underwent adult-to-adult LDLT were evaluated in this retrospective study [24]. The patients were divided into two groups: those who received oral supplementation with BCAAs before transplantation (BCAA group; n=129) and those who did not (non-BCAA group; n=107). Before the indication for LDLT was determined, BCAA supplementation was prescribed by a hepatologist to preserve hepatic reserve.

This strategy was carried out to delay a fatal reduction in hepatic reserve in patients with cirrhosis who were registered on a waiting list for liver transplantation. The administration of BCAAs to patients with acute liver failure was regarded as a contraindication. For preoperative oral BCAA supplementation, 86 patients took three packets of Livact BCAA granules (Ajinomoto Pharma, Tokyo, Japan) per day for more than 1 month before transplantation, and 43 patients took one to three packets of Aminoleban EN (Otsuka Pharmaceutical Co., Ltd., Tokyo, Japan) per day (50–150 g/day). The compositions of Livact and Aminoleban EN are compared in Table 2. The clinical characteristics and the incidence of bacteremia were compared between the two groups. With regard to clinical characteristics, the Child-Pugh scores (p=0.0003) and the model for ESLD scores (p=0.0008) were significantly higher in the BCAA group than in the non-BCAA group. The incidence of bacteremia for Child-Pugh class C patients was significantly lower in the BCAA group (6/90; 6.7%) than in the non-BCAA group (11/50; 22.0%, p=0.0132). In multivariate analysis, non-BCAA supplementation was an independent risk factor for bacteremia.

The reason that BCAA supplementation prevented bacteremia in this study [24] remains unclear. One possibility is improved nutrition for those suffering from malnutrition. In this study, there were no significant differences in body mass index and MUST scores (MUST was used as a screening tool for malnutrition in the BCAA and non-BCAA groups). Malnutrition has been reported to be common in patients with ESLD who are candidates for liver transplantation [25, 26]. Nevertheless, evaluation of malnutrition is extremely difficult in such patients [26-28].

Measurements of albumin and pre-albumin levels do not reflect nutritional status because hepatocellular protein synthesis is usually impaired in these patients. Assessment of a patient's body weight is difficult with the presence of ascites, pleural effusion, and peripheral edema. More objective measurements may be necessary for evaluation of the beneficial effects of BCAAs on nutritional status. Another possibility is that BCAA supplementation improves the immune system. Previous studies have shown the effect of changes in BCAA levels on the immune system. In previous cohort studies [29, 30], the BCAA supplementation groups showed elevated absolute lymphocyte counts. Bassit et al. reported that BCAA supplementation restored the ability of peripheral blood mononuclear cells to proliferate in response to mitogens after long-distance intensive exercise [31]. *In vitro* studieshave shown that omission of a single BCAA from medium of cultured lymphocytes completely abolishes protein synthesis and cellular proliferation [32-34].

Currently, few therapies are available for restoring immune activity, even in patients with liver cirrhosis. Nakamura et al. [20, 21] showed that phagocytic functions of neutrophils and natural killer activity of lymphocytes obtained from patients with liver cirrhosis were restored by oral supplementation with BCAAs.

Table 2. Comparison of the Compositions of Livact and Aminoleban EN

	Livact (4.15 g/Packet)	Aminoleban EN (50g/Packet)
Isoleucine (mg)	952	1922.5
Leucine (mg)	1904	2037
Valine (mg)	1144	1602
Gelatin hydrolysate (g)	-	6.5
Casein (g)	-	1.0
Carbohydrate (g)	-	31.05
Lipid (g)	-	3.5
Total energy (kcal)		210

Furthermore, Kakazu et al. [22, 23] demonstrated *in vitro* and *ex vivo* that an increased concentration of BCAAs restored the function of dendritic cells harvested from patients with cirrhosis. These findings suggest that BCAA supplementation can restore immune function in patients with advanced cirrhosis. Interestingly, Roth et al. [35] and Munoz et al. [36] showed lower levels of BCAAs in orthotopic liver transplant patients with sepsis.

The beneficial effects of BCAA supplementation on post-transplant bacteremia may reflect restoration of immune function. Previous studies have shown that BCAAs increase the absolute lymphocyte number count [31, 32], and for Child-Pugh class C patients in this study [24], the lymphocyte ratio tended to be higher in the BCAA group than in the non-BCAA group. This may partly explain the reduced incidence of bacteremia in the BCAA group. Preoperative oral BCAA supplementation may reduce the incidence of post-transplant bacteremia in LDLT patients. Further studies are necessary to better characterize the beneficial effects of BCAAs in LDLT patients.

Post-Operative Nutritional Support for Liver Transplantation

Liver transplantation has led to a significant improvement in nutritional deficiencies and metabolic disturbances evident in patients with ESLD. However, several factors, such as preoperative malnutrition, stress from surgery, and immunosuppressive therapy, enhance the need for nutritional support after transplantation.

In the last 2 decades, nutritional support has been recognized as a vital component for the management of critically ill patients, by delivering essential substrates, antioxidants, vitamins, and minerals, to aid patient recovery [37]. The advantages of enteral nutrition are well recognized, although the disadvantages of parenteral nutrition, particularly infectious and metabolic complications, have become evident [36, 37]. The significance of feeding across the small bowel in patients who cannot tolerate gastric feeding has also been recognized [38].

In our institution, Ikegami et al. [5] reported that early enteral nutrition was associated with a significantly reduced risk of developing bacterial sepsis after LDLT in the retrospective analysis of 346 adult-to-adult LDLT patients. The authors used enteral nutrition in LDLT via a transnasal feeding tube (New enteral feeding tube with a guide-wire, 10 Fr, Japan Sherwood Inc., Japan) and placed the tip of the feeding tube in the proximal jejunum. We routinely used enteral feeding within 12–24 hours. Enteral nutrition was started at 20 mL/hour for 12 hours and increased by 20 mL/hour every 12 hours to a maximal dose of 60 mL/hour. Patients given early intestinal nutrition were associated with a significantly reduced incidence of bacterial sepsis after LDLT. Moreover, the incidence of bacterial sepsis in patients starting enteral nutrition within 48 hours after operation was significantly lower than that of bacterial sepsis in patients starting enteral nutrition later than 48 hours.

The authors [5] explained that the intestine contains the largest bacterial flora in the body, and that the intestinal immune system and mucosal barrier system play important roles in protecting against bacterial infection [39-41]. Swartz and colleagues [39] reported that most of the pathogens isolated in patients with infectious complications after liver transplantation were derived from the intestine. Bacterial overgrowth and suppression of the intestinal antibacterial defense system are particular problems in patients with hepatic dysfunction, and are caused by portal hypertension, resulting in intestinal edema and decreased peristalsis [40].

Enteral nutrition could be effective in patients with such intestinal conditions. In fact, enteral nutrition has already been reported to stimulate bile flow and portal blood flow, prevent intestinal mucosal atrophy, and preserve intestinal structure and function [41]. Hasse and associates reported that, in patients undergoing LDLT, aggressive enteral nutrition decreased the incidence of bacterial infection from 29% to 14% [42]. Early enteral initiation of enteral nutrition after surgical or nonsurgical insults has been emphasized in recent years. Gianotti and coworkers [43] demonstrated that immediate enteral feeding in animals with burns was associated with a decrease in circulating stress hormones, increased gastrointestinal blood flow, and a reduction in bacterial sepsis.

Conclusion

Bacterial sepsis is one of the most lethal complications after LDLT. To prevent bacterial sepsis from developing, pre- and post-operative nutrition is a central issue for patients with liver cirrhosis after liver transplantation. Improved nutrition, including preoperative BCAA supplementation and early enteral nutrition, might support a functional immune system, and reduce septic morbidity and mortality in patients undergoing liver transplantation.

References

[1] Starzl TE, Groth CG, Brettschneider L, Moon JB, Fulginiti VA, Cotton EK, Porter KA. Extended survival in 3 cases of orthotopic homotransplantations of the human liver. *Surgery* 1968; 63 (4): 549-63.

[2] Starzl TE, Marchioro TL, von Kaulla K, Herrmann G, Brittain RS, Waddell WR. Homotransplantation of the liver in humans. *Surg. Gynec. & Obst.* 1963; 117:659.

[3] Starzl TE, Brettschneider L, Groth CG. Progress in transplantation. Copenhagen: Ejnar Munksgaards Forlag; 1967. *Recent developments in liver transplantation.*

[4] Harada N, Soejima Y, Taketomi A, Yoshizumi T, Uchiyama H, Maehara Y. Stenotrophomonas maltophilia bacteremia after living donor liver transplantation: Report of a case. *Surg. Today.* 2008; 38(5): 469-72.

[5] Ikegami T, Shirabe K, Yoshiya S, Yoshizumi T, Ninomiya M, Uchiyama H, Soejima Y, Maehara Y. Bacterial sepsis after living donor liver transplantation: the impact of early enteral nutrition. *J. Am. Coll. Surg.* 2012; 214(3): 288-95.

[6] Iida T, Kaido T, Yagi S, Yoshizawa A, Hata K, Mizumoto M, Mori A, Ogura Y, Oike F, Uemoto S. Posttransplant bacteremia in adult living donor liver transplant recipients. *Liver Transpl.* 2010; 16(12): 1379-85.

[7] Kim SI, Kim YJ, Jun YH, Wie SH, Kim YR, Choi JY, Yoon SK, Moon IS, Kim DG, Lee MD, Kang MW. Epidemiology and risk factors for bacteremia in 144 consecutive living-donor liver transplant recipients. *Yonsei. Med. J.* 2009 Feb 28; 50(1): 112-21.

[8] Rhee KW, Oh SH, Kim KM, Kim DY, Lee YJ, Kim T, Kim MN.Early bloodstream infection after pediatric living donor living transplantation. *Transplant. Proc.* 2012 Apr; 44 (3): 794-6.

[9] Hashimoto M, Sugawara Y, Tamura S, Kaneko J, Matsui Y, Togashi J, Makuuchi M. Bloodstream infection after living donor liver transplantation. *Scand. J. Infect. Dis.* 2008; 40 (6-7): 509-16.

[10] Man K, Lo CM, Ng IO, Wong YC, Qin LF, Fan ST, et al. Liver transplantation in rats using small-for-size grafts: a study of hemodynamic and morphological changes. *Arch. Surg.* 2001; 136: 280-285.

[11] Fondevila C, Hessheimer A, Taura P, Sånchez O, Calatayud D, de Riva N, et al. Portal hypertension: mechanism of injury and stimulus for

regeneration in porcine small-for-size transplantation. *Liver Transpl.* 2010; 16: 364-374.

[12] Ito T, Kiuchi T, Yamamoto H, Oike F, Ogura Y, Fujimoto Y, et al. Changes in portal venous pressure in the early phase after living donor liver transplantation: pathogenesis and clinical implications. *Transplantation* 2003; 75: 1313-1317.

[13] Man K, Fan ST, Lo CM, Liu CL, Fung PC, Liang TB, et al. Graft injury in relation to graft size in right lobe live donor liver transplantation: a study of hepatic sinusoidal injury in correlation with portal hemodynamics and intragraft gene expression. *Ann. Surg.* 2003; 237: 256-264.

[14] Kiuchi T, Onishi Y, Nakamura T. Small-for-size graft: Not defined solely by being small for size. *Liver Transpl* 2010; 16: 815-817

[15] Sanchez AJ, Aranda-Michel J. Nutrition for the liver transplant patient. *Liver Transpl.* 2006; 12:1310 -1316.

[16] Plauth M, Cabré E, Riggio O, Assis-Camilo M, Pirlich M, Kondrup J; DGEM (German Society for Nutritional Medicine), Ferenci P, Holm E, Vom Dahl S, Müller MJ, Nolte W; ESPEN (European Society for Parenteral and Enteral Nutrition). ESPEN Guidelines on Enteral Nutrition: Liver disease. *Clin. Nutr.* 2006 Apr; 25(2): 285-94.

[17] Malnutrition Advisory Group. A consistent and reliable tool for malnutrition screening. *Nurs. Times* 2003; 99: 26-27.

[18] Tietge UJ, Bahr MJ, Manns MP, Böker KH. Hepatic amino-acid metabolism in liver cirrhosis and in the long-term course after liver transplantation. *Transpl. Int.* 2003; 16: 1–8.

[19] Tsukishiro T, Shimizu Y, Higuchi K, Watanabe A. Effect of branched-chain amino acids on the composition and cytolytic activity of liver-associated lymphocytes in rats. *J. Gastroenterol. Hepatol.* 2000; 15: 849–859.

[20] Nakamura I, Ochiai K, Imawari M. Phagocytic function of neutrophils of patients with decompensated liver cirrhosis is restored by oral supplementation of branched-chain amino acids. *Hepatol. Res.* 2004; 29: 207–211.

[21] Nakamura I, Ochiai K, Imai Y, Moriyasu F, Imawari M. Restoration of innate host defense responses by oral supplementation of branched–chain amino acids in decompensated cirrhotic patients. *Hepatol. Res.* 2007; 37: 1062–1067.

[22] Kakazu E, Ueno Y, Kondo Y, Fukushima K, Shiina M, Inoue J, et al. Branched chain amino acids enhance the maturation and function of

myeloid dendritic cells ex vivo in patients with advanced cirrhosis. *Hepatology* 2009;50: 1936–1945.

[23] Kakazu E, Kanno N, Ueno Y, Shimosegawa T. Extracellular branched-chain amino acids, especially valine, regulate maturation and function of monocyte-derived dendritic cells. *J. Immunol.* 2007; 179: 7137–7146.

[24] Shirabe K, Yoshimatsu M, Motomura T, Takeishi K, Toshima T, Muto J, Matono R, Taketomi A, Uchiyama H, Maehara Y. Beneficial effects of supplementation with branched-chain amino acids on postoperative bacteremia in living donor liver transplant recipients. *Liver Transpl.* 2011; 17(9): 1073-80.

[25] Figueiredo F, Dickson ER, Pasha T, Kasparova P, Therneau T, Malinchoc M, et al. Impact of nutritional status on outcomes after liver transplantation. *Transplantation* 2000; 70: 1347–1352.

[26] Stephenson GR, Moretti EW, El-Moalem H, Clavien PA, Tuttle-Newhall JE. Malnutrition in liver transplant patients: preoperative subjective global assessment is predictive of outcome after liver transplantation. *Transplantation* 2001; 72: 666–670.

[27] Merli M, Giusto M, Gentili F, Novelli G, Ferretti G, Riggio O, et al. Nutritional status: its influence on the outcome of patients undergoing liver transplantation. *Liver Int.* 2010; 30: 208–214.

[28] Shahid M, Johnson J, Nightingale P, Neuberger J. Nutritional markers in liver allograft recipients. *Transplantation* 2005; 79: 359–362.

[29] Cerra FB, Mazuski JE, Chute E, Nuwer N, Teasley K, Lysne J, et al. Branched chain metabolic support. A prospective, randomized, double-blind trial in surgical stress. *Ann. Surg.* 1984; 199: 286–291.

[30] Vente JP, Soeters PB, von Meyenfeldt MF, Rouflart MM, van der Linden CJ, Gouma DJ. Prospective randomized double-blind trial of branched chain amino acid enriched versus standard parenteral nutrition solutions in traumatized and septic patients. *World J. Surg.* 1991; 15: 128–132.

[31] Bassit RA, Sawada LA, Bacurau RF, Navarro F, Martins E Jr, Santos RV, et al. Branched-chain amino acid supplementation and the immune response of long-distance athletes. *Nutrition* 2002; 18: 376–379.

[32] Chuang JC, Yu CL, Wang SR. Modulation of human lymphocyte proliferation by amino acids. *Clin. Exp. Immunol.* 1990; 81: 173–176.

[33] Dauphinais C, Waithe WI. PHA stimulation of human lymphocytes during amino acid deprivation. Protein, RNA and DNA synthesis. *J. Cell Physiol.* 1977; 91: 357–367.

[34] Waithe WI, Dauphinais C, Hathaway P, Hirschhorn K. Protein synthesis in stimulated lymphocytes. II. Amino acid requirements. *Cell Immunol.* 1975; 17: 323–334.

[35] Roth E, Mühlbacher F, Karner J, Steininger R, Schemper M, Funovics J. Liver amino acids in sepsis. *Surgery* 1985; 97: 436–442.

[36] Munoz SJ, Jarrell BE, Westerberg S, Miller L, Moritz MJ, Maddrey WC. Serum amino acids following human orthotopic liver transplantation. *Transplant. Proc.* 1993; 25: 1779–1782.

[37] Martindale RG, McClave SA, Vanek VW, McCarthy M, Roberts P, Taylor B, Ochoa JB, Napolitano L, Cresci G; American College of Critical Care Medicine; A.S.P.E.N. Board of Directors. Guidelines for the provision and assessment of nutrition support therapy in the adult critically ill patient: Society of Critical Care Medicine and American Society for Parenteral and Enteral Nutrition: Executive Summary. *Crit. Care Med.* 2009; 37(5): 1757-61.

[38] Heyland DK, Drover JW, Dhaliwal R, Greenwood J. Optimizing the benefits and minimizing the risks of enteral nutrition in the critically ill: role of small bowel feeding. *JPEN J. Parenter. Enteral Nutr.* 2002 Nov-Dec; 26(6 Suppl): S51-5; discussion S56-7. Review.

[39] Swartz MN. Hospital-acquired infections: diseases with increasingly limited therapies. *Proc. Natl. Acad. Sci. U S A.* 1994 29; 91 (7): 2420-7.

[40] Thalheimer U, Triantos CK, Samonakis DN, Patch D, Burroughs AK. Infection, coagulation, and variceal bleeding in cirrhosis. *Gut.* 2005; 54 (4): 556-63. Review.

[41] Moore FA, Moore EE. The evolving rationale for early enteral nutrition based on paradigms of multiple organ failure: a personal journey. *Nutr. Clin. Pract.* 2009 Jun-Jul; 24 (3): 297-304.

[42] Hasse JM, Blue LS, Liepa GU, Goldstein RM, Jennings LW, Mor E, Husberg BS, Levy MF, Gonwa TA, Klintmalm GB. Early enteral nutrition support in patients undergoing liver transplantation. *JPEN J. Parenter. Enteral Nutr.* 1995 Nov-Dec; 19(6): 437-43.

[43] Gianotti L, Nelson JL, Alexander JW, Chalk CL, Pyles T. Post injury hypermetabolic response and magnitude of translocation: prevention by early enteral nutrition. *Nutrition.* 1994; 10(1):32-6.

Index

B

C

D

E

F

G

J

K

L

M

N

O

P

Q

R

S

T

U